I Laughed So Hard
I Peed My Pants!

*A Woman's Essential
Guide for
Improved Bladder Control*

Kelli Berzuk
Physiotherapist

IPPC—Winnipeg, Manitoba, Canada

National Library of Canada Cataloguing in Publication

Berzuk, Kelli, 1968-
I laughed so hard I peed my pants! : a woman's essential guide for improved bladder control / Kelli Berzuk.

Includes index.
ISBN 0-9731841-0-8

1. Urinary incontinence--Popular works. 2. Urinary incontinence--Exercise therapy. 3. Women--Health and hygiene. I. Nova Physiotherapy & Sports Fitness Clinic. Incontinence & Pelvic Pain Clinic II. Title.

RC921.I5B47 2003   616.6'2   C2002-905938-0

Publisher & Distributor This book was published by IPPC—Incontinence & Pelvic Pain Clinic (division of Nova Physiotherapy & Sports Fitness Clinic)

714 Medical Arts Building, 233 Kennedy Street
Winnipeg, Manitoba, Canada, R3C 3J5
Phone: (204) 982.9178 Fax: (204) 982.9198

To James & Cassidy
my perfect little angels!

Book Cover Thank you to Ms. Charlene Kasdorf for the cover art work and Ms. Theresa Berzuk for the back cover text. My deepest gratitude to you both for your encouragement and guidance. Theresa, I will always appreciate the time and knowledge you offered so selflessly.

Illustrations Thank you to Mr. Kevin Gallays B.F.A., B.Ed. Your artistic talent and creativity was greatly appreciated.

Formatting Thank you to Ms. Sharon Caseburg, Production Editor—Turnstone Press. I will be forever grateful for your superb guidance and generosity in sharing your experience and wealth of knowledge.

Page Design Thank you to Ms. Corinne Gonen for all your hard work as well as your never ending support.

Dan Poynter Mr. Poytner's book, The Self-Publishing Manual, never left my side. This excellent resource walked me through the publication process, and made it a lot less intimidating. Thank you Mr. Poytner.

Printer Thank you to everyone from Friesen Printing in Altona, Manitoba, Canada. I would like to specifically thank Mr. Donovan Bergman, Mr. Gary Hamel, Mr. Ralph Hamm and Mr. Brad Schmidt for taking the time to answer my endless list of questions. Your patience and kindness was memorable.

Acknowledgements

This book would not have been possible without the help, guidance and dedication of many gifted individuals. I would like to extend my heart-felt appreciation to the following women and men who generously offered their time, special talents and support to bring this book to reality.

- Beverly Berzuk
- Theresa Berzuk B.Comm. (Hons.)
- Millie Braun M.Sc
- Corinne Dawley PHEc, B.H.Ec.(Nutr.)
- Erica Dyck
- Mireille Frechette B.ès. Sc., B.M.R.-P.T.
- Teresa Froese B.Sc(Hons.), MBA
- Corinne Gonen B.I.D.
- Tamara Hamin B.A., B.HEc., R.D.
- Lorraine Hilderman B.Sc Pharm.
- Julie Jerome
- Shelly Keast RN, BN
- Sarah Klassen B.A., B.Ed.
- Pat Lieblich B.P.T.
- Cynthia Markel Feldt M.P.T., A.T.C.
- Cheryl Martin B.Sc Pharm.
- Dorothy Plett
- Michelle Redekopp B.A., L.L.B.
- Karla Schultz B.A.
- Brenda Suderman B.J.(Honours), B.A.
- Anne Thornton-Trump M.L.S.
- Karly Vancott
- Penny Wilson B.S.R.
- Joseph Wong B.P.T., C.A.F.C.I.
- Chui Kin Yuen, MD, FRCSC, FACOG, FSOGC, MBA
  Chairman, Manitoba Clinic

The intent of this publication is to offer education regarding pelvic floor exercises to improve the overall health of the pelvic floor musculature, and to prevent or treat urinary incontinence. It is not meant to be a substitute for medical attention, but rather, can be most beneficial when used in conjunction with physician consultation. This self-help guide is not a replacement for medical care. Urinary incontinence may be a result of infection or other medical illness and therefore you should see your physician to discuss your symptoms. Medicine is a constantly advancing profession and new options are always being discovered. One of the treatment options for urinary incontinence is exercise. While many women benefit from proper exercise for their incontinence, some types of pelvic floor dysfunction require a physical assessment from a qualified health professional. As with all exercise, it is recommended you see your physician before commencing new exercise activities, especially when underlying medical conditions may exist.

Contents

Foreword

As a physiotherapist, dealing with muscle dysfunction and the painful effect it can have on individuals becomes a regular occurrence. Very quickly I gained respect for healthy and strong muscles and how they silently do their job, allowing us to go about our lives and activities without interruption. This changes instantly when someone experiences an injury.

In the pelvis there are muscles that also function in silence. The pelvic floor muscle holds the great responsibility of supporting your internal organs, increasing satisfaction in your sex life and preventing urinary and fecal leakage. This certainly is an important muscle! Amazingly, most of us do absolutely nothing to ensure its good health, and many do not even know it exists.

While muscle injury to the rest of the body usually produces pain and restricts function, thereby forcing people to seek medical attention, a weak or unhealthy pelvic floor muscle may have devastating effects that are rarely treated simply because help is seldom sought. At university in physiotherapy school, we briefly studied this muscle but, due to its internal location, our education and exposure to it was limited.

During routine physiotherapy assessments we would question patients on bowel and bladder leakage as an indicator of nerve injury. As a new graduate I was shocked to hear women answer repeatedly, **"Oh sure I leak when I cough or laugh, but that's normal."** They would often confess this with a slightly embarrassed laugh and then follow with, **"It is normal, isn't it?"** Well, I was not sure, but I needed to find out.

Since then, I have spent many years attending courses and conferences across North America regarding incontinence and pelvic floor muscle dysfunction, and I now work solely with patients experiencing problems specific to the pelvic floor musculature. In the past eight years, I have been fortunate to work with this special population of women and now what I repeatedly hear is; **"I wish I had known sooner that there was treatment for incontinence."** Well, now you will know how to help yourself!

While this book title tries to bring levity to the subject by using a phrase that many women identify with and quote frequently, I am compelled to remark that urinary incontinence is in no way a laughing matter. Loss of bladder control can inflict immense pain and devastating emotional consequence to the women affected as well as their loved ones. Sadly, it can diminish one's self-esteem and impede both social and physical activity. Thankfully, there is much that can be done to prevent and improve this situation. Most women show significant reduction or even resolution of their symptoms with simple home exercises and diet adjustments. Others who may have extensive weakness or damage to the pelvic floor musculature may require medical attention in addition to their home exercise program.

If you come across a section of text that has been noted in italics, this is a direct quotation. All indirect quotes will be distinguished simply by the superscript numeral. For further details, please see the references at the back of the book.

This book has been organized to provide introductory education on the functioning of the urinary system and the important roles of the pelvic floor muscle. It will then describe the common risk factors surrounding urinary incontinence before developing a proper home exercise program. I encourage you to read through the education component first in order to begin your strengthening program with a clear understanding of why improvement should be expected. Following the initial exercise component, additional practical steps for continued improvement will be presented, such as diet and lifestyle alterations, urge delay and relaxation techniques, and proper toileting postures. You will learn how to increase the intensity of your exercise routine to continually challenge yourself, and to incorporate exercise into your daily routine with the least interruption to your busy schedule. Finally, various treatment options will be discussed such as physiotherapy, pharmaceutical medications, bladder function testing and surgical techniques.

I hope you enjoy reading this book and have fun with the exercises while you customize them to fit your lifestyle. I know exercising can be frustrating at the beginning, but once you begin to regain bladder control and confidence, doing your exercises will become a simple and healthy part of your daily life.

Chapter 1: Introduction

You may be one of the millions of women experiencing episodes of lost bladder control, or perhaps you have watched others suffer and want to prevent this from happening to you. You may also be in the position where symptoms of bladder dysfunction have begun but you are not aware of these warnings signs. This self-help guide is important regardless of your current level of bladder control since a proper pelvic floor muscle strengthening program should be a part of every woman's life.

Recognize the Signs

It is vital to recognize voiding dysfunctions and urinary leakage early on so that you may stop the progression of these symptoms and work toward resolving the problem. Ask yourself the following questions:

- Do you refrain from laughing whole-heartedly?
- Do you cross your legs when you sneeze?
- Do you know the location of every washroom in your neighborhood?
- Do you use the washroom more than nine times a day?
- Do you leak urine when you cough, sneeze or exercise?
- Do you often have a strong urge to void (need to pee)?
- Do you race your children to the washroom?
- Do you need to reposition yourself on a chair until the feeling 'goes away' and then race to the washroom?
- Have you altered any physical or social activities because of decreased control over your bladder?

If you answer yes to any of the above questions, you may be experiencing urinary dysfunction and it is time to do something about it. Do not wait until these symptoms can no longer be hidden before you seek help. Improved bladder control is often attainable with a simple home program or with professional medical treatment.

Common Fallacies

Much more research is needed in the field of urinary incontinence to help us continue to develop better education, diagnostic and treatment protocols. We need answers to why one woman may be affected while another with similar birthing and medical history is spared. Even though we still have many questions requiring investigation, there are some common misconceptions that have been proven inaccurate. Three widely believed fallacies in the area of urinary incontinence are:

- Incontinence is a normal consequence of childbirth.
- Incontinence is a normal consequence of aging.
- Incontinence is something you just have to live with.

These statements could not be more wrong. Urinary incontinence is both preventable and treatable. Often improved diet and proper exercise is all that is needed to regain bladder control. Many patients are unaware that treatment is available and are often too embarrassed to talk to their doctor about it. This is very disturbing since most patients can be treated and dramatically improve their situation, often resolving their symptoms. If you are hiding the fact that you occasionally, or frequently, leak urine, it is important to know that many other women are living with the same problem. The goal of this self-help guide is to offer you the tools needed to regain control over your bladder. It is time to take a proactive approach to your bladder health in order to prevent or reduce urine leakage.

Key Points

- Millions of women in North America suffer from urinary incontinence.

- Incontinence can be prevented, treated and often cured with simple exercises and diet changes.

- Most women will not seek help or education due to embarrassment and the erroneous belief that nothing can be done about incontinence.

- It is time to take control over your bladder.

The following are terms commonly used by doctors, or seen in books and articles regarding incontinence.

Did You Know?

Dysuria (dis–yū'rē–ă) refers to pain or burning during voiding.

Nocturia (nok–tū'rē–ă) refers to the awakening from sleep because of a need to void.

Enuresis (en–yū–rē'sis) refers to urinary incontinence in children. This may be diurnal or nocturnal, that is urinary leakage may occur while awake or during sleep (bed-wetting) respectively.

Encopresis (en–kō–prē'sis) refers to fecal incontinence in children.

Nulliparous (nŭl–ip'ă–rŭs) refers to a female who has never borne children.

Multiparous (mŭl–tip'ă–rŭs) refers to a female who has given birth to more than one child.

Gravidity (gră–vid'i–tē) refers to the number of times that a female has been pregnant.

Parity (parĭ–tē) refers to the number of children to whom a female has given birth.

Chapter 2: Who Becomes Incontinent?

The Canadian Continence Foundation reports that:

- a 1997 study found 1.5 million Canadians suffer from urinary incontinence.[1]

The National Association For Continence (NAFC) reports that:

- 25 million Americans suffer from urinary incontinence.[2]

The Mayo Clinic web site estimates that:

- *half of all women in the United States experience urinary incontinence at some point in their lives.*[3]

In 2002 Pharmacia Canada stated that:

- approximately 2.9 million Canadians suffer from overactive bladder symptoms (urgency, frequency and/or urge incontinence) and less than 20% seek treatment.[4]

Recent studies in Europe and the American Nobel Study found that:

- previous estimates that 17 million Americans and 50 to 100 million people worldwide suffer from overactive bladder symptoms, may actually be understated.[5]

The Center for Bladder Control reports that:

- Of the 1.5 million residents in nursing homes, over
  50% are incontinent. Of the homebound elderly, 53% are
  incontinent.[6]

These unsettling statistics increase each year. Urinary incontinence is also greatly underreported because of the associated embarrassment. There are many reasons for urinary incontinence and anyone may be affected at any age. Boys and girls often have problems at night with bed-wetting, but many also display incontinence during the day. At night, decreased consciousness and a relaxed state play a large role, while during the day physical activity and giggling are common precipitants.

Between the ages of twenty and forty, women are more affected than men as a result of the stresses inflicted from pregnancy and delivery. Later in life, we see both men and women requiring treatment for incontinence. The hormonal fluctuation during menopause, combined with the physical change in bladder position, contribute to incontinence in women, while prostate changes are the common culprit for men.

The following is a typical scenario of a woman's experience with urinary incontinence:

A woman in her forties who has given birth to one or more children notices that she is leaking urine when she coughs, laughs, sneezes and exercises. At first she hopes the situation will resolve on its own, but as the symptoms begin to occur more frequently, the issue becomes increasingly difficult to ignore. Hiding from the problem usually leads to an increase in symptoms and may necessitate future surgery. The sooner this situation is addressed, the better. Unfortunately, she delays seeking medical attention until she experiences the very embarrassing situation of complete bladder emptying in public. This finally motivates her to discuss her problem with her doctor.

There is no reason for you to experience this stressful and embarrassing situation. Now is the time to see your doctor for a medical assessment and begin your home exercise program (see Chapter 12: Proper Pelvic Floor Exercises).

Another common scenario is the woman who has ignored the occasional leak over the years, assuming it is normal; her mother and grandmother both lost urine while laughing or coughing, as do most of her girlfriends. The common fallacy that urinary incontinence is a normal and acceptable part of aging and that nothing can be done to help anyway, supports her decision to start wearing a mini-pad daily and crossing her legs when she sneezes. She restricts her fluid intake and voids frequently in attempt to keep her bladder empty. Since her symptoms are 'not that bad' and easily hidden, she does not admit to herself that she has a problem with incontinence. This continues until she is hit with a bad cold leading to several days of intense coughing. This is the insult that puts her pelvic floor muscle over the edge. Her weakened and neglected muscle cannot tolerate the continuous stress of coughing and suddenly her rare dribbling becomes uncontrollable urinary leakage. This may all have been avoided with a proper exercise and education program.

It is important to know that while there are risk factors that increase your chances of losing control over your bladder, anyone may experience urinary incontinence. Social, economic or educational status are not factors in bladder control. Urinary leakage is something that women of all ages should be wary of, especially those planning to have children and those who have already given birth. Further research is needed to learn more about the underlying causes of urinary incontinence so that we may use this information to prevent a decrease in bladder control and to provide additional treatment options.

Since we are all susceptible to the life changes that contribute to urinary incontinence, it is vital that we keep our pelvic floor muscles as strong and healthy as possible. We need to be aware of diet and lifestyle factors that may lead to bladder instability.

On occasion, urinary incontinence may arise as a result of infection or other medical ailment. Discuss any problems with your family doctor to rule out underlying medical conditions.

Did You Know?

A study of 144 nulliparous (never given birth), female athletes ages eighteen to twenty-one, showed that 28% suffered from urinary incontinence. The breakdown according to sport specificity was as follows: 67% of the gymnasts; basketball players, 66%; tennis players, 50%; field hockey players, 42%; swimmers, 10%; volleyball players, 9%; softball players, 6%; and 0% of golfers studied experienced loss of bladder control. Interestingly, 40% of the incontinent female athletes reported urine leakage while involved in a high school sport, and 17% already had problems during a junior high sport.[7]

Physiotherapist's Viewpoint...

As a physiotherapist (referred to as physical therapists in the USA), I have treated bladder dysfunction in men, women and children from all walks of life. This book focuses specifically on female urinary incontinence. Throughout the following chapters I will be relating stories and experiences from some of the women I have been fortunate to learn from and treat. I hope you will find these anecdotes helpful as well as interesting. It is always reassuring to know that other women have similar symptoms and that you are not alone with this problem. It is even more important to know that most women improve or resolve their symptoms with simple exercise and diet alterations.

Patients often do not realize that they have a voiding dysfunction, at least not until they experience a major episode of leakage. You may gain insight to a potential problem when you enter a public washroom. Listen to other women in the stalls around you. How long do they urinate? Does their flow stop and start? In what ways does your void differ from or resemble voids of these women. As you read on, you will discover what is acceptable in a voiding pattern, and what is not. It will surprise you how many women do not have proper voiding patterns. These may be early warning signs of future urinary incontinence.

Key Points

- Urinary incontinence may affect any person of any age, culture or socioeconomic status.

- Women who have given birth are at an increased risk, but urinary incontinence also presents in women who have never been pregnant. It is no longer surprising to find young, athletic teenagers (especially those involved in high impact sports) who have problems with bladder control and they still have the pelvic floor stress of pregnancy ahead of them.

- It is important to keep your pelvic floor strong and healthy for the prevention of incontinence.

Did You Know?

It is very difficult to report the actual number of women suffering from incontinence. Research statistics range from 7% to 50% of females experiencing loss of bladder control at some point in their lives. Such variation in results may be due to the fact that many women do not offer this private information, while others may not even recognize the early symptoms of leakage. The social stigma and embarrassment associated with incontinence deters women from confiding in others, even their doctors, regarding their symptoms.

Overall, it is clear that millions of females worldwide experience urinary incontinence and symptoms of bladder dysfunction.

Chapter 3: Anatomy of the Urinary System

Before we can begin to address the problem of bladder dysfunction, it is important to have a simple understanding of how your urinary system works.

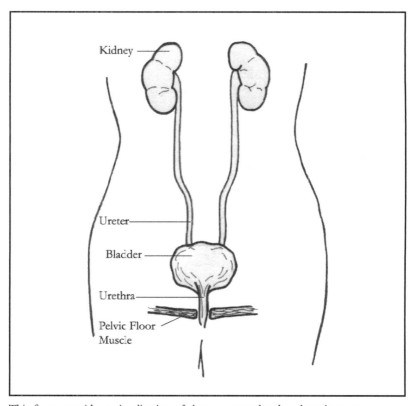

Kidney

Ureter

Bladder

Urethra

Pelvic Floor Muscle

This figure provides a visualization of the anatomy related to the urinary system.

The kidneys collect urine and then the urine travels through tubes called 'ureters' to the single urinary bladder. The urine sits in the bladder until we void or urinate (pee). From the bladder the urine exits the body by passing through a four cm (one and a half inch) tube called the urethra. Within the urethra there are sphincters or muscle rings (internal and external) that control the flow of urine.

The kidneys and ureters are considered the upper urinary tract, while the bladder, urethra and internal and external sphincters comprise the lower urinary tract. To be continent (to have full control of your bladder), you require a properly functioning:

- central nervous system and
- lower urinary tract.

Problems in the central nervous system require medical attention from your doctor. This book concentrates on dysfunction of the lower urinary tract and the pelvic floor musculature.

Phases of Continence

- Storage Phase
- Transition Phase
- Emptying Phase

Storage Phase

Your urinary bladder is a storage reservoir with a normal volume capacity of three hundred to six hundred milliliters (ten to twenty ounces). The walls of the bladder consist of a muscle known as the detrusor muscle. Embedded in this muscle are stretch receptors. These receptors are stimulated as the bladder fills and the walls of the bladder begin to expand and stretch.

The stimulated stretch receptors send signals to the brain, making you aware that you will soon need to void. The first desire to void begins at approximately 150 milliliters (four to five ounces) of filling.

The bladder remains relaxed until it reaches a volume of two hundred to 450 milliliters (seven to fifteen ounces); at that time the internal and external urethral sphincters, rings of muscle around the urethra, begin to contract harder to prevent urination.

The pelvic floor muscle makes up the external urethral sphincter and it is controlled by our conscious contraction of the muscle as well as the urethral-closing reflex that will be discussed in Chapter 4: The Nervous System. The internal urethral sphincter is controlled only by these reflexes.

Transition Phase

During the transition phase you voluntarily inhibit and postpone emptying of your bladder. Mental awareness is necessary to recognize the signals of fullness, leading to the decision that it is now time to find a washroom. Adequate mobility and dexterity are also required to transport you to a washroom. Women suffering with strong urge symptoms often notice a decreased length of time in this transition stage (see Chapter 18: Urgency & Urge Delay Techniques).

Emptying Phase

A person becomes very uncomfortable and must void at three hundred to six hundred milliliters (ten to twenty ounces). To empty the bladder, the detrusor muscle contracts while the pelvic floor muscle and urethral sphincters relax. This allows the urine to drain out of the bladder, through the urethra, and out of the body. Approximately fifty to seventy-five milliliters (one to two ounces) of urine will remain in the bladder after you finish voiding.

Key Points

• In the basic functioning of the urinary system, urine is collected in the kidneys, drains into the bladder via the ureters, and is removed from the bladder through the urethra. Urine travels down the urethra and exits the body.

• The internal and external urethral sphincters are important in preventing leakage of urine from the bladder. The pelvic floor muscle makes up the external urethral sphincter therefore we have control over the external urethral sphincter. The internal urethral sphincter is controlled by reflex messages.

• There are three phases in bladder function:

1. Storage Phase
2. Transition Phase
3. Emptying Phase

Did You Know?

Restricting your fluids will not decrease incontinence. In fact concentrated urine is irritating to the bladder (see Chapter 15: Bladder Irritants) and may lead to problems with urgency, the strong desire to void (see Chapter 18: Urgency & Urge Delay Techniques). As well, decreasing your fluid intake compromises bladder capacity and may lead to frequency, the need to void greater than nine times per day (see Chapter 17: Urinary Frequency). Fluid restriction may have promising short-term effects but devastating long-term results.

Notes

Chapter 4: The Nervous System

When discussing the role of the nervous system in bladder function, it is important to understand the involuntary reflexes (immediate messages) involved. The pelvic floor and bladder muscles work together but in an opposite fashion. As one contracts the other relaxes. This occurs by reflexes sent between the two muscles and is governed by our brain and nervous system. We need to appreciate this reflexive response so that we may take advantage of it when we try to calm our bladder urge (see Chapter 18: Urgency & Urge Delay Techniques), and to understand how a loss of these quick reflexes can lead to stress incontinence. During the bladder-filling phase, the bladder muscle should be relaxed to accommodate the increase in volume, while the pelvic floor muscle contracts to assist in closure of the urethra so that urine will not escape. As the bladder muscle expands, stretch receptors, located in the walls of the bladder, are triggered alerting us of the need to void.

While sitting on the toilet, we consciously relax our pelvic floor musculature. This sends a reflex message to our bladder muscle instructing it to contract. As the bladder contracts and begins to empty, urine fills the urethra. This triggers a separate reflex, from the urethra to the bladder, telling the bladder to contract even harder. We do not have to contract the bladder ourselves, the reflex does it for us. When the bladder is empty and the urethra notes that the volume of urine passing through it has decreased significantly, another reflex is triggered from the urethra to the bladder, instructing the bladder to calm down and stop contracting. As the bladder relaxes, a final message is sent from the bladder to the pelvic floor telling it to resume contraction to maintain closure while the bladder begins to fill again.

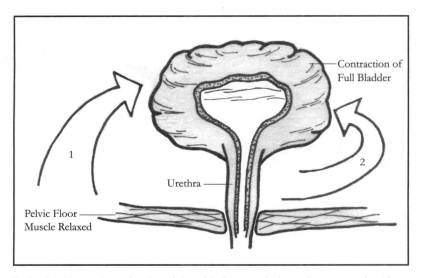

Reflex 1: With conscious relaxation of the pelvic floor muscle the urethra opens, and a reflex instructs the bladder muscle to begin contracting.

Reflex 2: As urine empties out of the bladder into the urethra, a second reflex is triggered instructing the bladder to contract harder.

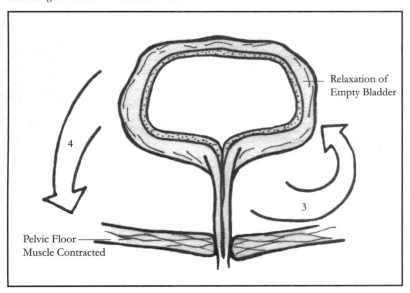

Reflex 3: As the urine flow into the urethra decreases (the bladder is almost fully emptied), a third reflex is triggered leading to relaxation of the bladder muscle.

Reflex 4: As the bladder muscle relaxes to begin the next filling stage, a fourth reflex instructs the pelvic floor muscle to contract and close the urethra.

This reflex system is of great significance for women suffering with stress incontinence. When we experience a sudden increase in pressure within our abdominal cavity (an increase in intra-abdominal pressure), there will be a resultant downward pressure on the bladder. For example, a split second before we sneeze or cough, our urethral sphincters squeeze the urethra closed and the pelvic floor muscle contracts to assist this closure. This is done to compensate for the sudden rise in intra-abdominal pressure. As the pelvic floor muscle contracts it sends a reflex message to the bladder telling the bladder to calm down and not push urine out.

Many events in life may dampen or damage this important reflex system. Nerve damage can occur with:

- bearing down during labor
- chronic constipation
- a chronic cough
- continuous heavy lifting at work
- the strain of being overweight

All will leave a pelvic floor at risk for damage to the nerves responsible for sending and receiving reflex messages. After injury by whatever means of stress or strain, you must work to reinstate this reflexive response. It follows the use-it-or-lose-it principle. All you need to do is start using it again (see Chapter 12: Proper Pelvic Floor Exercises). Just remember to tighten up this muscle before you cough, sneeze or lift heavy objects. After a while you will feel your pelvic floor contract without conscious control as you cough, sneeze and lift, and then you will know that you have your reflex back.

Key Points

- Reflexes between the bladder and the pelvic floor muscle can be lost if they are not used. Reinstating these reflexes is necessary for coordinated function between the bladder and the pelvic floor muscles.

- Understanding these reflexes gives us the tools to calm feelings of urgency (see Chapter 18: Urgency & Urge Delay Techniques) and reinstating these reflexes helps to decrease stress incontinence.

- Nerve damage may be a result of pregnancy and delivery, chronic straining, chronic coughing, repetitive heavy lifting, or being overweight. If the nerves supplying the pelvic floor musculature are damaged, incontinence may result.

Did You Know?

The first sensation of the need to void occurs at approximately 150 milliliters (four to five ounces) of bladder volume.

Chapter 5: Roles of the Pelvic Floor Muscle

The pelvic floor muscle is an extremely underrated and often neglected area of the body. Thankfully, it is also quite resilient and forgiving. It takes only a small amount of consideration and exercise for this muscle to respond positively. It is often injured with pregnancy, vaginal delivery, constipation, the strain of a chronic cough, or the effects of obesity. In spite of all these common methods of injury, the pelvic floor muscle is rarely given even the slightest amount of attention.

Now is the time to recognize the significant contribution made by the pelvic floor muscle and to promote its protection through strengthening.

The pelvic floor musculature has three very important functions:

- Sphincteric
- Supportive
- Sexual

Sphincteric

The pelvic floor musculature assists in closure of the urethral and anal sphincters. This means that the urethral and anal openings will have a more complete closure when the pelvic floor muscle is strong and healthy. The proper closing of these openings is imperative for the maintenance of continence, both urinary and fecal. If the pelvic floor musculature does not function adequately in closing the urethral and anal openings, incontinence may result. The following chapter will address several types of urinary incontinence that may be experienced.

Supportive

The pelvic floor musculature is responsible for supporting the internal pelvic organs. The stronger the musculature, the less likely it is that you will experience prolapse. Chapter 7 will describe the different types of pelvic organ prolapse.

Sexual

Laxity or weakness in the pelvic floor muscle may decrease sexual appreciation and sensation. Chapter 8 will look at the role of the pelvic floor musculature in sexual satisfaction.

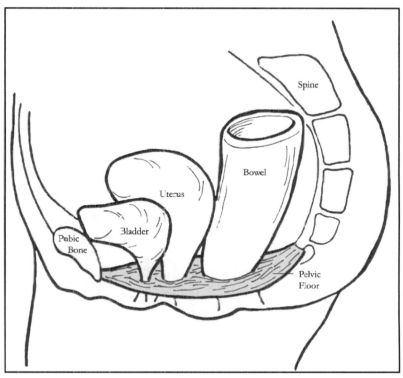

The pelvic floor supports the pelvic organs and contributes to sexual sensation and closure of the bladder and bowel.

Key Points

- The pelvic floor muscle is responsible for three very important functions; sphincter closure, support of the pelvic organs, and sexual appreciation. Our lives would be significantly disrupted if any of these responsibilities were not met.

- Common stresses invoked daily on our pelvic floor may be chronic coughing, straining with constipation or simply being overweight. These can leave the muscle at risk of injury.

- Very few women work at keeping their pelvic floor healthy to ensure proper function. Exercise of the pelvic floor rarely begins until after it fails to do its job. Thankfully, the pelvic floor muscle is resilient and very forgiving.

Did You Know?

Progesterone during menstruation combined with muscle swelling leads to a temporary decrease in muscle strength and coordination. This is why women tend to have more incontinence and feelings of heaviness in our pelvis with PMS.

Chapter 6: Urinary Incontinence

Urinary incontinence is the involuntary loss of urine (in any amount, from a few drops to complete bladder emptying), or the inability to control when and where emptying of the bladder will occur. Loss of bladder control may be occurring for different reasons and therefore there are several types of urinary incontinence.

Stress Incontinence

Stress incontinence is the involuntary loss of urine when the pressure within the abdomen exceeds the pressure within the bladder. For example, activities such as laughing, coughing, sneezing, lifting, running, jumping and aerobics will increase the pressure in the abdomen and pelvis and press on the bladder (some women even report leakage with a hiccup). This may force urine out of the bladder and urethra. Picture yourself pressing on the outside of a water balloon. If the knot was unable to hold the neck of the balloon shut, the water would begin to dribble or pour out. Strengthening our pelvic floor muscle is like tightening up the 'knot' on the urethra.

Stress incontinence may result from muscle weakness and laxity, pregnancy and delivery, pelvic surgery or injury, and/or menopausal and hormonal changes.

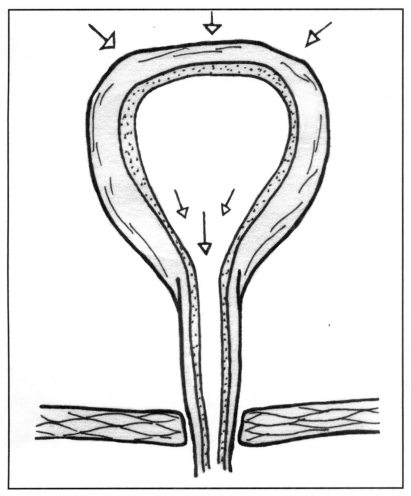

A sudden increase in abdominal pressure pushes urine out of the bladder. The weakened pelvic floor muscle is unable to close off the urethra and leakage results.

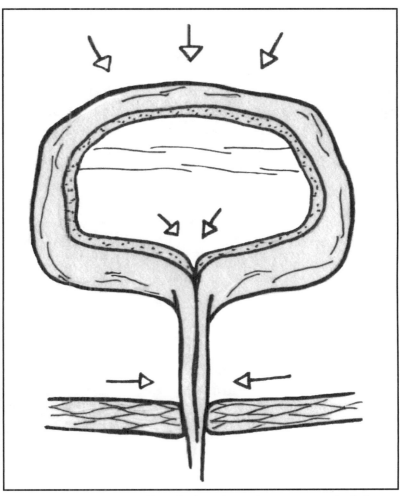

A strong pelvic floor muscle effectively closes the urethra to prevent urine leakage when intra-abdominal pressure rises suddenly.

Urge Incontinence

Urge incontinence is the involuntary loss of urine associated with a strong desire or urge to void. In this circumstance, a person is aware of the need to empty their bladder but will often leak before reaching the toilet. The bladder muscle begins to contract and eliminates the transition phase that would normally allow us the time needed to locate a washroom.

Urge incontinence is often triggered by hearing water running, becoming cold or wet, or simply unlocking the door to your house. This last problem is so common that it is often referred to as the-key-in-the-door syndrome. As you approach the safety of your home and washroom, even though you have had no warning sensation of a need to void, suddenly your bladder begins to involuntarily contract and empty before you reach the washroom.

For women, urge incontinence may result from bladder instability, estrogen hormone changes, bladder irritants, or certain pharmaceutical medications. For men, urge incontinence is often the result of prostate enlargement.

It is important to note that urge, or the strong desire to void, may be present with or without urinary incontinence. Daily strong urge may be an indicator of bladder dysfunction even when leakage is not a problem.

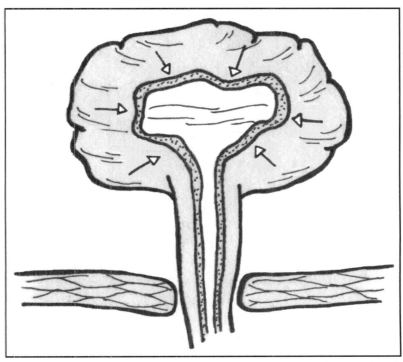

Irritation of the inside bladder lining leads to contraction of the bladder muscle and the intense feeling of urgency.

Mixed Incontinence

Mixed incontinence is simply a combination of both stress and urge incontinence. Often women notice initial symptoms of stress incontinence that, when left untreated, develop into urgency symptoms and mixed incontinence.

Functional Incontinence

Functional incontinence is the involuntary loss of urine due to mental impairment or physical restrictions. This is often seen in the elderly who may have limitations in being able to get to the washroom or self-toileting. Often a consultation with an Occupational Therapist can resolve this problem.

Women experiencing functional incontinence should ensure that there is a clear pathway to the washroom and that they wear clothing that is easily removed. These women may also benefit from following a voiding schedule, perhaps voiding every three hours, to prevent accidents. Some women find it helpful to monitor their pattern of needing to void, use this information to create a voiding schedule, and then go to the washroom at these pre-determined times. A caregiver may need to assist with toileting. It may help to post pictures of a toilet throughout the house as prompts to go to the washroom when there is no caregiver present.

Overflow Incontinence

Overflow incontinence is the involuntary loss of urine when an over-distended bladder cannot be fully emptied. This is often associated with disorders of the nervous system. Medical intervention and catheterization are treatment options for patients experiencing overflow incontinence.

This book focuses on the first three types of incontinence; stress, urge and mixed incontinence, since these are often associated with changes in the pelvic floor musculature.

Physiotherapist's Viewpoint...

There are many reasons for encouraging women to seek medical help. The following are a few examples of what I see clinically.

Hiding the Signs

Often women begin leaking occasionally when laughing, coughing and sneezing. This continues to progress gradually over the next few years, while they struggle to ignore and hide the problem. Some women start to wear a mini-pad daily, while others refuse to give in to their demanding bladder. Women will usually adjust their activities, perhaps dropping their aerobic class, or becoming increasingly aware of the location of every washroom around them. Some women even say that they try not to laugh too much; I still find this comment very unsettling to hear. Just imagine the control the bladder has on their quality of life; it can even affect their sense of humor!

It is fairly common for women to initially try to ignore the fact that they are incontinent. They frequently become quite creative in finding ways to hide their symptoms while they suffer in silence. Their social world gets smaller, activities less frequent, and black becomes a standard color of clothing.

Slowly they may experience the beginning sensations of urgency. Often they will compensate for this by restricting their fluid intake and voiding more frequently to keep their bladder empty. As their bladder shrinks in volume and their urine becomes more concentrated, the urge and frequency **increase**. The vicious cycle continues.

By this point women are often consumed with thoughts of their bladder. They consider their urinary leakage before making vacation plans, before playing tag with their children, and while socializing with friends.

The Flood

The final straw comes when they experience the most embarrassing situation of all, a flood. Many women recall such an event; it is usually a special evening that ends in humiliation. The following is a common scenario:

She was dancing with her husband, relaxed and having a wonderful time. They had a nice dinner earlier, with wine and coffee, and were enjoying their rare, romantic night together. Suddenly the strong feeling of bladder urgency consumed her and this was immediately followed by complete bladder emptying, in public and on her beautiful dress.

I have heard similar stories over and over again. Women recount their embarrassment with tears and horror. Some women have experienced this flood at work, others while playing golf. It can happen anywhere. I remember one woman relating her episode of flooding while singing a solo at the front of church.

After these embarrassing situations, women usually realize that they are no longer able to hide their incontinence symptoms and that it is time they do something about the problem. Most women see their family doctor while others research the Internet for information. Every woman should see a doctor, either her family doctor or a gynecologist, for a medical assessment to rule out possible infection or underlying health problems.

It is always easier to rectify the problem sooner rather than later, but it is **never** too late to start.

Long Standing Incontinence

The first year that I began treating female urinary incontinence, all of my referrals were for women over the age of seventy-five. Most had undergone multiple bladder lift surgeries and had been leaking for twenty to forty years. I remember reading the referrals and wondering if treatment would be worth their effort.

I am happy to report that these remarkable women very quickly put my worries to rest. They were gutsy and determined to improve. Some had given birth five times or more, some had experienced decades of urinary leakage, while others had undergone surgery, bladder lifts and often a hysterectomy. These experiences granted them a much better understanding of the pelvic floor than I had at that point. Thankfully, they were very generous and patient in sharing their knowledge with me.

What a thrill it was for me to see their intense motivation when given the tools to help themselves. They were sponges for education and a proper exercise protocol.

I had pre-judged these women with concerns that they may be uncomfortable discussing their pelvic floor since they had been raised in a more conservative era. I also incorrectly believed it may be difficult for them to remember to do their exercises, and even wondered if there was any hope for improvement after such extensive pelvic floor damage.

In eight short weeks of treatment each of these women showed a 60 to 100% improvement.

The education I gained was invaluable, and I will always be grateful to these women. They taught me that it is never too late to treat a motivated woman, regardless of age or how long the problem has been present.

Preventing Incontinence

Several years into my Women's Health practice, I received my first physician referral requesting patient education in the prevention of urinary incontinence. This piece of paper brought joy to my heart. What a turn around; women were now becoming aware of the shocking prevalence of female urinary incontinence and wanting to take a pro-active approach to ensuring that their pelvic floor would always be healthy and strong.

Exercise to Enhance Surgical Results

Another memorable day for me was the first time a surgeon referred a patient for pelvic floor strengthening pre- and post-surgery. This surgeon advised his patient that the stronger the muscles, the more successful and longer lasting the results of the surgery would be. This surgery was a hysterectomy due to severe uterine prolapse. The day after surgery this patient gently resumed her pelvic floor exercises. She gradually increased her exercise program over the next few months. The exercises were not difficult for her since she had developed her routine pre-surgery and therefore was already comfortable locating the correct muscle and fitting the exercises into her day. I am happy to report that she experienced no incontinence post-hysterectomy.

The next pre-surgery referral I received was for a bladder lift. This patient worked very hard and, when the surgeon saw her three months later, both doctor and patient were very pleased with her progress and decided to cancel the surgery.

Key Points

- One of the three major functions of the pelvic floor is to close off the urethral and anal sphincters to prevent urinary and fecal leakage.

- Stress and urge incontinence, or a mixture of both, are types of urine leakage associated with the functioning of the pelvic floor musculature, and are often experienced by women. Urinary incontinence often begins as stress incontinence and, when left untreated, develops into urge incontinence as well.

- It often takes the humiliation of a flood to encourage women to seek help to correct the problem.

- Simple pelvic floor exercises can improve bladder control (regardless of age or length of time that symptoms have been present), may prevent the necessity of surgery, and can augment the results of surgical repair.

Did You Know?

If incontinence has caused skin irritation or rash, the following tips may be helpful:

- Wear 100% cotton underwear only.
- Wash your underwear with gentle soaps rather than detergent.
- Rinse well and do not use fabric softeners.
- Instead of pantyhose, wear stay-ups or a garter belt with hosiery.
- Avoid bubble baths and bath oils.
- Avoid using soap when washing your perineal area, lots of water is best.
- Avoid using tampons since they may cause urethral or bladder irritation.
- Never use vaginal deodorants or douches.

Chapter 7: Pelvic Organ Prolapse

As previously mentioned, the pelvic floor muscle has three main functions; sphincteric, supportive and sexual. We will now look at the second objective of the pelvic floor muscle; support. When the pelvic floor muscle is weak, it may not effectively support the pelvic organs, such as the uterus, the urinary bladder, the urethra, the rectum, and the small intestines. The word *prolapse* means falling down. When these organs sit lower than their standard positions, prolapse can occur. Often your doctor will assign a grade to your prolapse depending on the severity. There are many grading systems used to objectify the degree of the prolapse. The following are some commonly reported symptoms of pelvic organ prolapse:

- feeling of heaviness in the perineum (area between legs)
- pelvic pressure
- feeling of 'falling out'
- lump in the vagina
- lump in the rectum
- discomfort with intercourse
- pelvic or low back pain
- difficulty defecating completely
- constipation
- urinary incontinence
- urinary retention (difficulty emptying bladder completely)
- urinary urgency
- urinary frequency (having to urinate frequently)

These symptoms usually increase in severity later in the day and after prolonged standing. During the initial stages, many women with pelvic prolapse experience no symptoms, and are unaware of any organ descent until it is detected by a physician during a routine pelvic examination.

There are many different types of pelvic prolapse since one or more of several organs may be affected. As well, the prolapse is named according to the pelvic floor opening that the organ is protruding into: the vagina or the anus. The following is a description of several types of prolapse that are commonly seen:

Cystocele

A cystocele is the backward and downward bulging of the urinary bladder into the vagina. When the front wall of the vagina is not appropriately supported, symptoms such as urinary stress incontinence or urinary retention may arise. If urine is not able to fully empty out of the bladder, it becomes an attractive area for bacteria to grow and this may lead to recurrent urinary tract infections (bladder infections).

Cystoceles may become a problem following hysterectomy. This is due to the change in support. The bladder can no longer rely on the uterus to keep it pushed forward and as a result, the bladder may now fall backward into the vagina.

Urethrocele

A urethrocele is the downward and backward descent of the urethra into the vagina. As with a cystocele, this may also have a significant effect on the urinary tract, depending on the severity.

Uterine Prolapse

A uterine prolapse is the downward displacement of the uterine cervix into the vagina. Women who are breast-feeding should note that the decrease in hormone production during nursing could aggravate uterine prolapse. For this reason, pelvic floor muscle exercise is especially important at this time.

Enterocele

An enterocele is the descent of the small intestine down the back vaginal wall. This lack of support may lead to difficulty with bowel movements and may result in constipation.

When the uterus is removed, the small intestines tend to relocate into the now empty position. With poor support, the intestines may then fall downward into the vagina.

Rectocele

A rectocele is the forward and downward displacement of the rectum into the back vaginal wall. As with an enterocele, this may produce problems with defecation. As well, the resultant constipation and straining will further increase the stress on the pelvic floor muscle, and may displace the rectum further. Remember that chronic straining will also increase the risk of urinary and fecal incontinence.

Rectal Prolapse

A rectal prolapse is the rectum descending through the anal opening. It is often mistaken for, or confused with, a hemorrhoid. This again may produce difficulty with bowel movements. A diet high in fiber and adequate fluid intake will help to keep stool soft and thereby decrease the need to strain with defecation (see Chapter 15: Bladder Irritants).

Did You Know?

In 1999, gynecologist Dr. Bob L. Shull, estimated that 43 million American women, over the age of 65, will experience some degree of pelvic organ prolapse by 2030.[8]

Physiotherapist's Viewpoint...

Not long ago I saw a patient referred for treatment of a uterine prolapse and urinary incontinence. The prolapse was very significant and this patient had to push her uterus back into her vagina several times each day. The patient reported significant discomfort by the end of her workday, as well as irritation of the cervix itself. She was not a surgical candidate because of a serious medical condition.

She spent several months trying to increase the strength of her pelvic floor but, unfortunately, she was showing very little improvement despite her great effort.

Her family doctor then arranged for her to be fitted for a pessary, which is an orthotic device used to support a woman's uterus (see Chapter 24: Available Treatment Options). This was quite effective in supporting the falling tissue, but still did not decrease the urinary incontinence. She continued her home exercise program and within a few weeks of using the pessary she began showing improvement in muscle strength. Once the pressure of the prolapse was lifted from her pelvic floor, the exercises became effective. A few months later, this patient had improved from her initial five to ten leakage episodes per day, to one to two leaks per week.

Key Points

- The second major function of the pelvic floor is to support the pelvic organs within the pelvis.

- In some women the bladder, uterus, rectum or intestines may prolapse, or fall downward with gravity, due to a lack of support.

- Since a prolapsed uterus is the reason many women require hysterectomy, it is important for all women to keep their pelvic floor muscle strong and provide the necessary uterine support.

Did You Know?

Women with a cystocele may have to stand up after voiding and then sit down again to fully complete urination. Always try to reposition your body, lean forward and shift side to side, if you think that your bladder may not be fully emptied.

Chapter 8: Sexual Function

The pelvic floor musculature consists of several muscles, with the most significant one being the pubococcygeus muscle. This muscle is located in the deepest layer of the pelvic floor and is responsible for the sexual sensation felt by women as well as their partner. More superficially are the bulbospongiosus and ischiocavernosus muscles. The function of these muscles is to arouse the clitoris in women and the penis in men. They also contribute to the rhythmic contraction during orgasm.

These muscle groups should be thought of as one muscle and will be exercised and strengthened as a single entity. Throughout this book these muscles will be grouped together and referred to as the pelvic floor muscle.

As in the walls of the bladder, the pelvic floor muscle contains stretch receptors. When the muscle is stretched, the receptors stimulate nerve endings, and this triggers sensation. A healthier muscle will have more bulk or tone and will therefore stretch to a greater extent. As the stretch increases, greater stimulation occurs to the nerve, and the result is an increase in sensation experienced. As the pelvic floor muscle increases in strength and tone, an overall increase in sexual satisfaction may be noted.

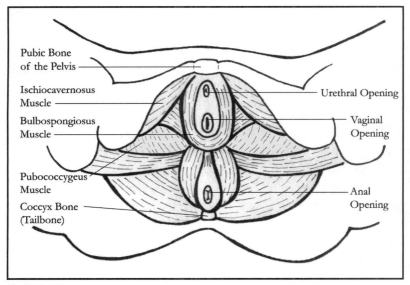

Pubic Bone
of the Pelvis

Ischiocavernosus
Muscle

Bulbospongiosus
Muscle

Pubococcygeus
Muscle

Coccyx Bone
(Tailbone)

Urethral Opening

Vaginal
Opening

Anal
Opening

This inferior view shows the muscles that make up the pelvic floor.

A Combination of Symptoms

The three functions of the pelvic floor, sphincteric, supportive and sexual, are performed simultaneously. This is why a weakened or unhealthy muscle may result in a combination of symptoms such as pain with sexual intercourse, or urinary leakage during intercourse. A dysfunctional pelvic floor may fail in one or more of its three very important roles.

Patients with pelvic organ prolapse may experience discomfort or even pain during sexual intercourse. If you are experiencing this symptom, you may notice that as the strength of the pelvic floor increases with exercise, there is a gradual decrease in discomfort. In the meantime you may want to try different sexual positions. Remember that gravity pulls the organs downward; therefore, lying flat will probably be more comfortable than sitting or standing.

For a muscle to be healthy it must be able to relax as well as contract. To perform these movements well, a muscle requires a good blood supply and therefore lots of oxygen delivery. Patients with too much tension in their pelvic floor musculature, such as many vulvodynia (chronic vulvar discomfort usually described as burning, stinging, irritation or rawness to the region) patients for example, can have great pain with intercourse. A healthy pelvic floor muscle will be strong, providing closure and support, as well as greater sexual sensation. It will also have the ability to relax and therefore be less prone to painful muscle spasm and hypertension.

Urinary leakage during sex is also a common concern. On occasion, as arousal begins, the pelvic floor muscle relaxes and a few drops of urine may leak out. This again should become less of a problem as your muscle becomes stronger. Be reassured by the fact that a man rarely notices when a woman leaks urine during intercourse. Even though this may be a consuming thought in your mind, it is probably not what is going through his. Do not let this concern prevent you from engaging in sexual relations.

Occasionally, women report full bladder emptying during intercourse. This flooding is usually experienced on penetration, if bladder contraction is triggered, or during orgasm, when involuntary relaxation occurs. Strengthening your pelvic floor may help with these problems; however, you should see your physician to investigate the cause of your symptoms. Also talk to your sexual partner about your concerns. You may have difficulty discussing the subject, but it could be a long-term problem and you and your partner will need to work through it together. In most cases women are surprised at the supportive response they receive from their partners.

You may also want to take this opportunity to gain feedback from your partner. Try a few pelvic floor contractions (see Chapter 12: Proper Pelvic Floor Exercises) during sexual intercourse and see if your partner notices an increase in strength.

Again, have fun and enjoy the benefits of all of your exercises. Remember that sex is a workout in itself for your muscle. Your body will be tired so do not do your pelvic floor exercises immediately after sex or you will be using a fatigued muscle. Rest and relax; your exercises can wait for a few hours.

Pelvic Pain Syndromes

As previously mentioned, being able to properly relax your pelvic floor and having a healthy muscle may play a key role in the prevention of pelvic pain syndromes. While this book concentrates on female urinary incontinence, the main objective is the overall health of your pelvic floor. It is therefore important to be aware that many women suffer greatly with vulvar, vaginal and bladder pain that is often related to sexual intimacy. These pain conditions may also be treated with pelvic floor muscle exercises in conjunction with treatment by medical disciplines such as gynecology, urology, urogynecology, family medicine, psychology and physiotherapy.

There is research suggesting that women who as children experienced day or nighttime incontinence may be at greater risk of pelvic pain syndromes in their adult lives. Use this information as a warning to ensure that your pelvic floor is healthy and strong and to seek help and education to prevent these problems. If you suffered from urinary problems as a child, then you will have further motivation to exercise your pelvic floor musculature.

Physiotherapist's Viewpoint...

I would like to end this chapter with a story of a remarkable woman who touched my heart and is truly an inspiration, especially to other women who have been affected by pelvic pain. This was one of my first experiences in the treatment of pelvic pain dysfunction, and I am grateful to this woman for all that she has taught me.

This woman was referred to our clinic with a diagnosis of vulvodynia that had begun on her honeymoon, five years previous. During her first sexual experience she knew that something was very wrong since she felt extreme pain with intercourse. She sought medical attention and tried medication, surgery and counseling. She noted some improvement but was still suffering with vulvar pain. By the time I met her, she and her husband had given up the hope of having children and their marriage was strained. Intercourse was infrequent and difficult for both of them; eventually they avoided it all together.

I was honored to be included in her team of physicians and psychologists, but at the same time terrified that I would have nothing to offer her. Her referring doctor informed me that by this point in her dysfunction, the pelvic floor muscle was involved and might now be a major contributor to her pain.

We began treatment and realized very quickly that her extreme pelvic floor muscle tightness and spasm was in fact a direct link to her pain.

Over the next year she worked diligently and made outstanding progress. Her wonderful husband was very supportive and their counseling with a chronic pelvic pain psychologist was going well. I remember when she confided in me that she was actually able to enjoy intercourse with her husband for the first time; this was an amazing breakthrough for them.

Toward the end of her treatment, I asked her not to return until she and her husband had sexual intercourse three times. As a joke, she asked me to write this down as a prescription. Well imagine my surprise when she returned to the clinic two days later. Further treatment was not indicated. Two years later they were blessed with a precious baby.

Key Points

- The third role of the pelvic floor is sexual function.

- It is equally important for a muscle to have a strong contraction as it is for it to have the ability to fully relax.

- When the pelvic floor muscle is unable to contract sufficiently, it may result in a decrease in sexual satisfaction. When a muscle cannot fully relax, it may lead to pelvic pain or discomfort during intercourse.

Did You Know?

Many women with incontinence report that it has affected their work and social relationships.

Chapter 9: Factors Related to Incontinence

There are many factors that increase your chances of experiencing loss of bladder control at some time in your life. The most common ones are listed below.

- Pregnancy
- Vaginal delivery
- Diastasis recti
- Aging
- Medication
- Recurrent urinary tract infection
- Being female
- Childhood incontinence
- Family history of incontinence
- Menopause/hormonal changes
- Increased weight
- Hysterectomy
- Pelvic floor surgeries
- Abdominal surgeries
- Chronic constipation
- Chronic cough
- Diet containing bladder irritants
- Smoking
- Radiation therapy
- Diseases such as: Alzheimer's, Diabetes, Multiple Sclerosis and Parkinson's Syndrome

Some of the greater risk factors will now be explored. If you are at risk, then it is important to begin a preventative program immediately. If you work on addressing the risk factors within your control, and begin your pelvic floor strengthening program, then you will improve your chances of avoiding incontinence throughout your lifetime. Use this as a wake-up call; you do not have the luxury of neglecting your pelvic floor.

Pregnancy & Vaginal Delivery

Among the most notable factors contributing to female urinary incontinence are pregnancy and labor. This is not to say that women who have never been pregnant, or have never had a vaginal delivery, do not experience loss of bladder control. Women without offspring, as well as men and children, can also suffer from incontinence, yet it is most common in women who have given birth.

Pregnant women are notorious for constantly running to the bathroom. Frequency (the need to void more than nine times in a day) is a symptom expectant mothers joke about constantly. It is easy to understand why this occurs, since their fluid intake must increase to accommodate the baby's needs and blood supply.

Frequency during pregnancy often goes hand-in-hand with the very annoying bladder symptom of nocturia. This is the experience of being wakened from sleep because of the need to void. Nocturia occurs because of the increased intake of fluid that is often not fully eliminated during the day. The pressure of the baby impedes circulation in the legs and, when lying flat, the fluid is able to flow to the kidneys and urine is produced. It may be helpful for pregnant women who suffer with nocturia to decrease their fluid intake two to three hours before going to sleep, as well as to lie down and elevate their legs one to two hours before bed. This will allow the fluid in their lower extremities to flow to their kidneys and then be eliminated as urine, hopefully before falling asleep.

Urgency is also a complaint during pregnancy. Pregnant women often feel that their baby must be sitting on their bladder. Any pressure on the bladder wall can stimulate the stretch receptors of the bladder muscle and therefore send false messages to the brain, erroneously telling the bladder that it is full. This will be further explored in Chapter 18: Urgency & Urge Delay Techniques.

With these urinary symptoms often comes loss of bladder control. Stress, urge or mixed incontinence can occur in any or all of the trimesters of pregnancy. Women who experience leakage during pregnancy may continue to have problems after delivery. The best method of preventing these problems is to combat these new stresses with a strong pelvic floor muscle. It is never too late to start your exercises, but the earlier the better. Going into pregnancy with an already strengthened muscle is the best scenario, and continuing your exercises during pregnancy and post-partum gives your body the resources for preventing the loss of bladder control.

Many women have concerns that a strong pelvic floor muscle may contribute to difficulty during labor. This could not be more wrong. A strong and healthy muscle has the ability to give an effective contraction, as well as fully relax. These functions are equally important during a vaginal delivery.

When it is time for the baby's head to engage, the pelvic floor will assist in turning and guiding the baby through the birth canal. A healthy muscle will contract as needed and then relax to open, when appropriate. By ensuring that this muscle has proper strength and endurance, you will better support the baby during pregnancy and then promote better muscle function during delivery.

If you are one of the lucky ones who do not have any bladder problems during pregnancy, you may not be out of the woods. There are many reasons that incontinence is seen post-partum. Damage to soft tissues may occur during delivery. Injuries may include strain, stretching and even tearing of the pelvic floor musculature, connective tissues, ligaments and nerves. This in turn can affect support of the bladder and urethra. Damage to the pelvic floor musculature may decrease its effectiveness in assisting the urethral sphincters in closure.

The nerves that supply these muscles may be stretched or torn during delivery. The pudendal nerves and pelvic nerves (that supply the bladder and pelvic floor musculature) are positioned on either side of the birth canal and are therefore at risk of injury. These nerves carry messages to the pelvic floor muscle and the bladder, and it is important that the nerves remain healthy for proper message transfer and subsequent continence post-partum.

Forceps or vacuum suction may be used in assisting delivery of the baby and these devices may also affect the muscles, nerves, ligaments and connective tissue. The size of the baby is also significant; larger babies often cause more injury.

Another factor that may contribute to incontinence post-partum is the fluctuation in hormone levels. Relaxin is a hormone that circulates through the body and promotes laxity of joint ligaments. This hormone is necessary for delivery of the baby and may take up to six weeks to be fully eliminated from the body. During this time the pelvic floor musculature may not contract efficiently and therefore be unable to effectively close the urethral sphincters.

Also notable is the decrease in estrogen levels during breast-feeding, when ovulation temporarily ceases. Estrogen is needed for proper closure of the urethral sphincters.

Whether or not you experience urinary or fecal leakage following the birth of your baby, remember that damage to your pelvic floor musculature has been done. If you do not make a conscious effort to rebuild its strength and endurance as well as reinstate the urethral-closing reflex to respond to any sudden increase in intra-abdominal pressure, then you are setting yourself up for loss of continence sometime in the future. Your next chest cold, a sudden heavy lift, the birth of your next child, menopausal hormone changes, an increase in body weight or simply the passage of time, could put your pelvic floor musculature over the edge. Any new stress on the pelvic floor may trigger the beginning of leakage.

This chapter is not meant to scare you, but rather to impress on you what your body must go through when you carry and deliver a baby. When you are aware of the facts, you can make informed decisions. The pelvic floor takes a beating with pregnancy and delivery, and it is time to start respecting the important functions of this muscle. Mothers will give up anything for their children, but they do not necessarily have to give up their bladder control. Thankfully the pelvic floor muscle is very forgiving, and a little exercise goes a long way.

Pelvic floor exercises may be started twenty-four to forty-eight hours after the birth of your baby. Begin gingerly and gradually progress to your pre-delivery exercise program. With your new, amazingly busy schedule and never-ending demands, all compounded by sleep deprivation, you may need to rely on reminders to do your exercises. Refer to Chapter 14: Red Dot Program.

Rest for twenty-four to forty-eight hours, you deserve it. Afterwards, very gently contract your pelvic floor muscle a small amount, even if you have stitches. Continue to try to achieve minimal muscle contractions. This is important to begin blood circulation and encourage healing to this area. As fresh, oxygenated blood moves in, inflammation will be pushed out. Over the next few days, increase the intensity of your contraction, within your tolerance.

Some women find heat or ice to the perineum helpful to decrease pain and swelling and promote blood flow. Remember that your sensation to hot and cold may be altered, so ensure that you have a wet towel wrapped around the ice pack, or that the water in a tub or water bottle is not overly hot. An ice pack or hot pack may be used for up to twenty minutes, several times per day.

During your much dreaded, post-partum bowel movement, give your exhausted and battered perineum some support. The bowels will empty at the back of your pelvic floor and there is no reason to put strain on the middle and front sections of the muscle. Use your hand, toilet paper roll covered with clean tissue, or a sanitary pad to lift and support the front half of your perineum. This action will protect your pelvic floor muscle as well as make your bowel movement less uncomfortable.

If you need to cough or sneeze, use your hand or pillow to support the perineum. This again is to save your pelvic floor and to decrease discomfort. It is crucial that you tighten up your pelvic floor every time you increase your intra-abdominal pressure since your pelvic floor will be unable to protect itself. If, understandably, you cannot effectively contract your muscle yet, then support it any way you can. Your hand or a rolled up towel work well.

By about day five to seven post-partum, you should try to resume your pre-delivery exercise program of pelvic floor exercises. Again, do this within your tolerance, and gradually increase the intensity and hold time of your contraction, as well as the number of repetitions.

Remember, when you are breast-feeding, your hormone levels will prevent your pelvic floor muscle from reaching its full potential. It will take time for your nerves and muscle fibers to heal and resume their normal function. Be patient if your contraction feels weak; the strength will resume over time.

Did You Know?

Incontinence is **not** a normal consequence of childbirth.

Diastasis Recti

Diastasis recti is a medical condition where the rectus abdominus muscle of the abdominal wall is split. This is most commonly associated with pregnancy but can occasionally be found in children, men and also women who have never been pregnant. Obesity and chronic lung disease can also be contributing factors to this condition.

It is important to mention diastasis recti because when the center of the abdominal wall exhibits this lengthwise separation, it can no longer provide good support to the internal organs. This allows the pelvic organs to rest heavily on the pelvic floor, leading to interference in proper contraction of the pelvic floor muscle and therefore may cause or increase urinary incontinence. For assessment or treatment of this condition see your physician or physiotherapist. Physiotherapists can offer exercise advice on how to reduce or control the diastasis.

Did You Know?

In 1995, Dr. Teh-Wei Hu at the University of California-Berkely found the total costs related to urinary incontinence in the US was approximately $27.9 billion for the sixty-five and older age group. The breakdown was as follows:

Routine Care, $10.2 billion; Longer Hospital Stays, $6.2 billion; Urinary Tract Infections, $4.2 billion; Home Care, $4.2 billion; Additional Admissions, $1.6 billion; Treatment, $667 million; Diagnostic Tests, $390 million; Skin Care, $380 million; and Falls, $58.4 million.[9]

Aging

There are numerous changes to the pelvic floor with age, and unfortunately, each impact the muscle's ability to properly function. Some of these changes are as follows:

Hormonal Changes

Hormonal changes during menopause affect continence for many women. The decrease in estrogen levels can affect proper closure of the urethral sphincters, since the bladder neck and urethra become thin and more brittle. The estrogen changes will also leave the bladder muscle itself in a leathery state, less able to contract fully, and more prone to muscle spasms and urgency (see Chapter 18: Urgency & Urge Delay Techniques).

Estrogen is also responsible for proper blood circulation. As the flow of blood decreases, blood vessels and the tissues of the urethral wall will begin to flatten, causing the diameter inside the urethra to enlarge. This leads to poor closure of the urethra since as estrogen concentration decreases, the urethral sphincters may no longer close as effectively, and it is additionally challenged as the urethral tube widens and requires more, not less, closing strength. The decline in estrogen and resultant decrease in blood circulation also impedes the strength and efficiency of the pelvic floor muscle and its ability to effectively assist in urethral closure. Muscles thrive in areas of good blood flow and oxygen delivery and become less healthy when not well nourished.

Estrogen also keeps collagen fibers healthy. As the estrogen levels drop, the collagen fibers may not be able to support the urethra effectively in its proper position.

A decrease in estrogen will affect the cells that line the inside of the bladder and produce a thinning, less elastic bladder wall. This can leave the bladder more easily affected by a bladder-irritating diet and lifestyle.

The nerves carrying messages to the bladder are also affected by a change in estrogen production. Less estrogen will increase the sensitivity in the nerve and may trigger problems with bladder muscle spasms and urgency.

Chronic Cough or Constipation

If you have suffered with a chronic cough for many years, perhaps secondary to smoking or a lung disorder such as asthma, then it can be expected that the years of sudden increases in intra-abdominal pressure will have weakened your pelvic floor. Chronic constipation and years of straining will have added further damage to your pelvic floor. Most likely you were unaware of the need to combat these stresses with pelvic floor strengthening exercises. If you have not exercised your pelvic floor muscles, then there will be atrophy of the muscle. Atrophy is the loss of muscle bulk that follows the use-it-or-lose-it principle.

With an increase in age often comes a decrease in bowel movements and constipation. As activity levels slow down and food consumption decreases, so does the movement within the intestines. This change in digestion can produce more straining and therefore damage to the pelvic floor muscle. It is very important to increase fiber, and fruit and vegetable consumption as well as participate in some form of exercise such as daily walks, to prevent constipation.

Decreased Mobility

With age often comes a decrease in mobility. This may be due to arthritis or other joint pain and medical ailments. This limit on mobility may hinder the speed and ability that physically gets you to the washroom. It may also lead to an increase in weight, that could then promote urinary incontinence. When you finally reach the washroom, arthritic hands can make it difficult to open zippers and remove your clothes.

Alteration in Perception of Signals

Aging may also cause a decrease in awareness of the messages that warn you of the need to void. There is often a reduction in response time because of the decreased recognition of the signals, as well as the bladder muscle being more easily irritated and therefore contracting more frequently. For example, the elderly often find the sound of running water is enough to trigger the sensation of needing to urinate. This, along with a decline in physical speed, may affect bladder control.

Changes of the Bladder Muscle

As we age, the strength of our now 'leathery' bladder muscle will diminish, reducing its ability to contract. This may lead to incomplete bladder emptying. The size of the bladder decreases in capacity leading to frequency in urination. Often this is accompanied by an increase in nighttime urine production and needing to void several times at night. This mixed with medications such as diuretics (water pills), or other medical ailments, such as high blood pressure or neurological disorders (Alzheimer's, Diabetes, Multiple Sclerosis and Parkinson's Syndrome), can greatly compromise bladder control. Medications for other medical conditions can decrease the contractility of the bladder muscle, decrease the bladder's ability to stretch and hold the normal urine volume, or drugs can also interfere with the urethral sphincter's ability to close off the urethral.

Overall, it is easy to see that life will challenge our bladder control with each phase of maturity. We need to be prepared to meet these challenges, and it is surprisingly easy to do. It is never too late to start exercising and almost everyone sees improvement in bladder control as the result. Some will see complete resolution of symptoms, while others will gain differing degrees of control. The sooner you start the better, but it is never too late.

Did You Know?

The second leading reason for institutionalization in the elderly is urinary incontinence.[10]

Incontinence is **not** a normal part of aging.

Medications

Loss of bladder control may occur as a result of some medications. Drugs necessary for the treatment of medical conditions often have side effects, and it is not uncommon for these side effects to include bladder symptoms such as urgency or incontinence. If you feel that a drug may be contributing to urinary leakage **do not** alter your medication plan. Speak to your physician or pharmacist; another drug may be available that will not have this bladder effect and still meet your medical needs. If there are no other pharmaceutical options, then it is up to you to do all that you can to combat these side effects. Altering your diet, losing weight, and strengthening your pelvic floor and surrounding muscles can often decrease the amount of leakage, even when it is medication induced.

The following commonly used medications may negatively affect bladder function:

Decongestants, beta-blockers (some examples include propranolol, metoprolol and atenolol) and calcium channel blockers (some examples may include amlodipine, felodipine, diltiazem, nifedipine and verapamil) may promote urinary retention by increasing

urethral sphincter tone and decreasing bladder contractility.
This may lead to overflow incontinence (see Chapter 6: Urinary
Incontinence for a definition of overflow incontinence) and
frequency.

Antidepressant, antihistamine, antiparkinson, antipsychotic
and antispasmodic drugs may also lead to urinary retention by
decreasing bladder contractility and therefore promote overflow
incontinence. Decreased awareness and impaired mobility may
further amplify poor bladder control.

Alpha-adrenergic drugs (doxazosin, prazosin and terazosin)
that are often used in the treatment of high blood pressure or
benign prostate hyperplasia may decrease internal sphincter tone
and therefore affect continence.

Diuretic medications (hydrochlorothiazide and furosemide)
may increase urgency and frequency.

Psychotropic and sedative drugs may cause over-sedation,
confusion, and immobility that impair your ability to get to the
washroom and may affect response time and comprehension of
bladder signals.

Recurrent Urinary Tract Infections

Urinary tract infection (UTI) is a medical concern that requires
physician attention and often antibiotic treatment. Another
name for recurrent UTI is cystitis where 'cyst' means bladder
and 'itis' means inflammation. Women may also suffer from
urethritis, referring to inflammation of the urethra.

Both of these problems can lead to instability of the bladder.
Medications usually clear up the infection; however, it is
sometimes difficult to resolve the inflammation of the bladder
lining. These tissues are swollen, hot and now produce pain when
urine touches the bladder lining. This irritation to the bladder
causes it to contract in an attempt to eliminate the burning urine.
This produces the very strong urge to void, even if you have
just tried to empty your bladder a few minutes earlier. To relieve

the symptoms, immediately increase your water consumption to dilute your urine and therefore decrease the irritation. Avoiding bladder irritating foods and beverages, as listed in Chapter 15: Bladder Irritants, will also aid in healing.

Common symptoms of UTI are:

- Frequency with little urine output
- Urgency
- Burning
- Pain with urination
- Low back pain
- Low abdominal pain
- Blood in urine
- Fever
- Chills

By keeping your pelvic floor muscle strong, it can assist in closure of the urethra. This is important not only for keeping urine in, but also for keeping germs out and thereby preventing infection. A strong healthy muscle will promote a good blood supply to the region, and this helps the body to fight off infection and disease.

Did You Know?

Incontinence can lead to emotional disturbances and social isolation.[11]

Incontinence can have a significant impact on self-esteem.

Key Points

- If any of the common bladder control risk factors pertain to you, then you need to take a pro-active role in prevention.

- Pregnancy and labor, aging, hormonal changes and medications are very important risk factors to be aware of.

Did You Know?

You should urinate five to nine times each day with two and a half to four hours between voids, except during pregnancy or when breast-feeding.

Chapter 10: What Can I Do for Myself?

It may be hard to believe, but you could be peeing incorrectly. Many women have picked up bad habits over the years. Appropriate voiding behaviors and possible bladder irritants will be discussed in the following chapters so that you may alter any incorrect peeing problems. You will be provided with the tools required to begin and maintain an effective home exercise program to strengthen your pelvic floor and normalize bladder control. For information regarding medical advances used to prevent or decrease incontinence and bladder dysfunction, see Chapter 24: Available Treatment Options.

Did You Know?

Chinese Proverb: The bladder is the mirror of the soul.

Physiotherapist's Viewpoint...

One of the many wonderful things about my patients with urinary incontinence is their excitement when given the tools to help themselves. Physiotherapists treating general musculo-skeletal injuries often spend much time encouraging patients to do back or neck exercises. Since I began focusing my practice on this special population of pelvic floor dysfunction, I have had the refreshing change of, occasionally, holding women back from their daily exercises. These patients try so hard that, at the beginning, they may do exercise excessively and fatigue their pelvic floor muscle. Start off slowly and allow strength and endurance to build gradually.

Key Points

- A proper exercise program, diet changes and correct voiding techniques are all areas that you have the ability to alter. You can improve your diet and bladder habits, and complete your daily exercise routine in the privacy of your home and without anyone knowing.

- Correction in these areas can significantly reduce or eliminate urinary incontinence for many women.

- You have more control over your symptoms than you may realize.

Did You Know?

Incontinence is **not** 'just something you have to live with'.

Chapter 11: Why Exercise a Muscle?

As we begin exercising a muscle, the initial effect will be an increase in vascularity (blood flow). This improvement in blood supply is necessary for greater oxygen delivery that in turn will produce a healthier muscle. As exercise continues, proper oxygenation leads to a more fit muscle.

A second benefit will be the development of muscle memory. The body is amazing: once you have sent a message along a nerve pathway to a particular muscle, to either contract or relax, the muscle will remember this response. Efficiency in passing messages from nerve to muscle or muscle to nerve will continue to improve from this point on. Just as you never forget how to ride a bike, a muscle does not forget how to contract. Once the muscle has learned, it will continue to build on this information.

A muscle is made up of many small sections called motor units. A weak muscle has only a few motor units contracting. As a muscle gains strength, more motor units start to work. It is important to get them all working together. As a well structured exercise program continues, you will benefit from getting more of the motor units within a muscle to contract together. You will see larger sections in the muscle being used and in a more coordinated fashion.

Finally, after months of diligent exercise you will benefit from hypertrophy of the muscle. Hypertrophy is the increase in the size of the muscle. Over time an enlargement of each individual muscle fiber diameter can be measured. As each fiber thickens, the muscle as a whole will bulk up. This will not be noticeable in the size of the pelvic floor muscle, but rather in an increased strength of the muscle.

These muscle developments will occur in stages as will the objective improvements. Chapter 23: Signs of Regaining Bladder Control, discusses this further. As mentioned previously, the benefits specific to exercising the pelvic floor musculature are these:

- Improved bladder control,
- Improved bowel control,
- Prevent or reduce pelvic organ prolapse, and
- Improve sexual satisfaction.

Key Points

- Benefits seen in a properly exercised muscle: improved blood supply, better use of oxygen, increased efficiency in transferring information between the nerve and muscle, and thickening of individual muscle fibers within a muscle.

- Exercise of the pelvic floor muscle is to improve sexual sensation, bladder and bowel control and prevent prolapse.

Did You Know?

The Agency for Health Care Policy and Research, U.S. Department of Health and Human Services (formerly AHCPR, now known as AHRQ; Agency for Health Care Research and Quality) reported that the annual medical cost for urinary incontinence care totaled $16.4 billion, $11.2 billion in the community and $5.2 billion in nursing facilities.[12]

Chapter 12: Proper Pelvic Floor Exercises

The purpose of this guide is to promote bladder health for women. This is achieved by taking a pro-active approach in the prevention of urinary incontinence or in trying to regain control once symptoms have begun. Realistically most women will not seek out instruction on how to properly exercise their pelvic floor until they have already experienced some decrease in bladder control. While this may be unfortunate, it is never too late (or too soon) to start.

Goals of Pelvic Floor Exercise

The goals of the following daily exercise program are first to improve the pelvic floor muscle strength to prevent urine loss, and second to regain the urethral-closing reflex. As discussed in Chapter 4: The Nervous System, the urethral-closing reflex allows a quick contraction of the pelvic floor when there is a sudden increase in intra-abdominal pressure. This may happen with a cough or sneeze. This is why women with stress incontinence will want to work on regaining their closing reflex.

You will also want to ensure that your urethra-closing reflex is working efficiently if you suffer from urge or mixed incontinence so that you may overcome inappropriate bladder muscle contractions. When your bladder is irritated it may begin to contract when it should be relaxed, as when drinking caffeinated coffee. As the bladder muscle begins to contract, the pelvic floor musculature should quickly contract via the urethral-closing reflex and in this way prevent leakage. Both an increase in strength and efficiency of the urethral-closing reflex will be necessary to regain control over your bladder.

Position

To begin your exercises, lie on your back in a quiet room. It may be difficult to locate and contract this muscle if it is very weak, as is often the case, so it is important to be in a place where you will be able to relax and focus. Remove yourself from all distractions, such as the television or children requiring your attention. Some women like to dim the lights or play relaxing music. Place two pillows, or a stool, under your knees. This will allow you to relax more fully. This will also help to reduce the pull of gravity on the muscle you want to contract. This is important since at this point you will want to make the exercise as simple as possible.

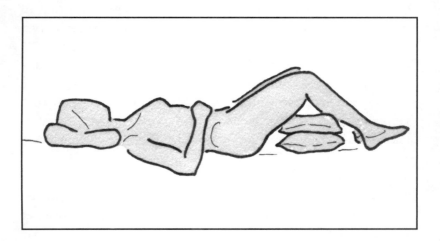

Breathing

Next concentrate on your breathing. Resist holding your breath or clenching your teeth while doing these exercises. Relax. When you hold your breath you will deprive your muscles of the much needed oxygen. Holding your breath also causes contraction of your abdominal muscles and this produces an unwanted, downward pressure on the pelvic floor.

Try to breathe in during relaxation and breathe out during muscle contraction. This will allow the lungs and the pelvic floor muscles to work together instead of having the lungs pushing downward, as the pelvic floor muscle is trying to lift upward.

Isolate Your Pelvic Floor Muscle

Initially much concentration is required to isolate the pelvic floor muscle. Focus on the muscle that you use to stop the urine flow when voiding, or to hold back gas in a crowded elevator.

Relax your Abdominals

Find the muscle and contract. During this time your abdominals, or tummy muscles, should be completely relaxed. When you are tightening your pelvic floor muscle you should be pulling them up and in. When you contract your abdominal muscles you will be pushing down and out, through the pelvic floor. It will make it more difficult to tighten your pelvic floor when your abdominal muscles are not relaxed. Place your hand lightly on your lower abdomen to ensure that your tummy muscles do not tighten as you contract your pelvic floor. If this happens, stop, relax, and try again.

If you are finding it difficult to relax your abdominal muscles while doing your pelvic floor exercises, try getting down on the floor on your hands and knees. Put a cushion by your head and rest on your forearms, from elbow to hand. This will tilt your head downward and decrease the pull of gravity on your pelvic floor. Now let your tummy muscles sag toward the ground. Try your pelvic floor contractions from this position and see if it is easier to isolate the correct muscle, without contracting your abdominals.

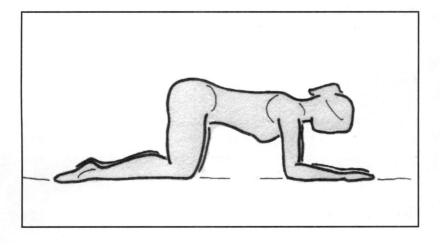

Relax your Gluteals

Remember to relax your gluteal muscles as well. These are the large muscles that make up your buttocks. Your hips and legs should be relaxed. If you are clenching your gluteal muscles, then you are using the wrong muscle. If your body lifts up and off of the ground when you are lying on your back, then you are probably using your gluteal muscles. The pelvic floor muscle is located between the left and right buttock and is not capable of raising your body upward.

Relax your Hip Adductors

Should you see your knees pressing together, then your hip adductors (groin and inside thigh muscles) are contracting. This again is the wrong muscle to contract. It is fine if your knees lightly rest against each other, but your legs should not be squeezing together.

If you see your body moving, then you are probably using the wrong muscle. When you contract your pelvic floor, no one around you should be able to tell that you have done this exercise.

Double-Rest Period

Once you are able to locate the muscle between your legs that stops urination and the passage of gas, concentrate on making a visual image of it. If you have never exercised this muscle before, start off very slowly and increase gradually. For example, contract the muscle for three seconds and then rest for six seconds. You will want to rest, or relax the muscle for twice as long as you contracted. This will help to prevent fatigue of the muscle. This double-rest period is only required for the first few weeks of your exercise program. As endurance builds you may decrease your rest period to equal your hold time. Some people may even be able to contract their long hold contractions for six or seven seconds. If this is the case for you, then you do not need to use a double rest period. There is no need to rest longer than ten seconds because it will take too long to complete your exercises.

Two Types of Exercises

There are two methods to do your pelvic floor exercises;

I. Long Hold Contractions
II. Quick Contractions

The difference between these two exercises is that you will contract the same muscle for differing lengths of time.

I. Long Hold Contractions

1. It is a good idea to begin a program customized to your present abilities. Count how many seconds that you are able to hold the contraction. If you can hold for one to two seconds, for example, then strive to make your program a three to four second hold. Always set your goal one or two seconds greater than what you are capable of doing.

2. Now that you have decided how long to hold the contraction, double this number for your rest period. For example, your three-second hold will be followed by a six-second rest period.

3. Next you need to decide how many times to repeat this contraction. If you can easily feel your contraction, you may choose to make your goal one to two repetitions greater than

the number that you can easily complete. For example, if you think that you are able to properly complete the contraction three times then aim for four or five repetitions to build up your muscle strength.

Long Hold Contractions

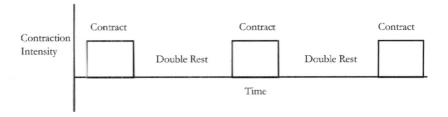

Customized Long Hold Contractions

If you can easily feel the length of time you are able to hold and the number of repetitions you are able to complete, you may choose to customize your exercise program. If you find that you are able to hold your contraction for two seconds and you can do three contractions before your muscle becomes tired, then you may decide that your home program should be the following;

- **Contract three seconds.**
- **Rest six seconds.**
- **Repeat four times.**
- **This equals one set.**
- **Complete ten sets spread throughout each day.**

Sample Long Hold Contractions

If you are unsure how long you are holding the contraction, or how many repetitions you can properly execute, then start with the following sample exercise program. This pre-set program will be less confusing for counting. Hold your contraction for five seconds and then rest for a count of ten seconds. Repeat five times. This exercise regime is appropriate for most people. If you find that it is too difficult or too easy, then you should be following the customized program.

For simplicity, many women choose the following;

- **Contract five seconds.**
- **Rest ten seconds.**
- **Repeat five times.**
- **This equals one set.**
- **Complete ten sets spread throughout each day.**

Your goal will be to complete fifty contractions each day, holding for five seconds, and resting for ten seconds. This may sound like it will be very time-consuming however, it really is not since each of the ten sets will only take approximately one minute to complete.

Splitting Up the Sets

Whether you choose the sample or customize your own program, you will want to complete ten sets of exercises spread throughout the day. Again, this is to prevent muscle fatigue. For example, you may want to complete three sets in the morning, four sets before dinner and three sets before bed. This may sound like a lot of exercise but remember each contraction takes only a few seconds and less then a minute to complete a set.

You may split them up even further. Some women choose to do two sets, five times a day. I have even asked women with very low muscle endurance to perform one set each hour to complete ten sets without causing muscle fatigue. For most women this may not be a realistic goal. It is hard enough to remember to do your exercises two or three times in the day, ten times is often impossible.

Adjust the program to suit your day, keeping in mind that your muscle will fatigue quickly. For example, if you were to do all ten sets at the same time, only the first few sets would be done well. If you start your exercise program using the correct muscle and then notice that you have begun to use your abdominal (tummy muscles), gluteal (buttocks), or hip adductor (squeezing your knees together) muscles, then you have fatigued your pelvic floor muscle and are incorporating these accessory muscles to do the work. If this is the case, stop and rest. **It will be counterproductive to continue exercising as you have already worked your pelvic floor to fatigue.**

II. Quick Contractions

In addition to your long hold contractions, you will need to do quick contractions. For these you simply squeeze your pelvic floor muscle tightly and then immediately let go and relax. You should hold the contraction for approximately one-second, rest one second, and repeat.

It is important to do both types of exercises since muscles are made up of two different types of muscle fibers. The pelvic floor musculature consists of 85% of fibers that react slowly but also fatigue slowly. The remaining 15% of the muscle fibers consist of a fiber type that uses a separate oxygenation process and therefore can react much faster but then quickly fatigue. By completing both the long hold and quick contractions, you will ensure that all fibers of the muscle are being strengthened.

Test your quick contractions and count how many you are able to do before fatiguing. If you can do three, then aim for four quick contractions per set. Again, you will complete ten sets throughout the day. To make counting easier, many women match the number of repetitions of quick contractions to the number of long hold contractions they are doing. If you are doing five long hold contractions, follow this with five quick contractions. Often women find the quick contraction the easier of the two exercises. Just remember to let your muscle relax fully before starting your next quick contraction. You may have to rest one to two seconds between each quick contraction.

Quick Contractions

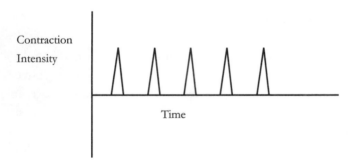

Complete Sample Exercise Program

If you have chosen the sample program rather than customizing your own, then the following is a good exercise program to keep the numbers simple to count.

I. Long Hold Contractions:

- **Contract five seconds.**
- **Rest ten seconds.**
- **Repeat five times.**

II. Quick Contractions:

- **Contract one second.**
- **Rest one second.**
- **Repeat five times.**

This is one set of each type of exercise. To allow the muscle fibers a greater resting period, you should alternate between each type of exercise, one set of long hold contractions, and then one set of quick contractions, etc.

It will take approximately one minute to complete one set of each of the two exercises (long hold and quick contractions). Remember you will need to complete ten sets of each every day. As previously mentioned, you may choose to complete three sets of both types of exercise in the morning, four sets of each before dinner, and your final three sets before bed. Try to adjust this routine to fit easily into your day, this way it will be the least inconvenient to your busy lifestyle. Again, do not tighten your abdominal, gluteal or hip adductor muscles or hold your breath during either type of contraction.

Exercise Progression

As your exercises become easier you will want to increase the level of difficulty of your program to further challenge your pelvic floor muscle. Exercises may be progressed in the following three areas.

1. Change Position

In the beginning, all exercises should be done in the same position: lying on your back with your knees bent and your feet slightly apart. You may want to slide pillows or a stool under your knees. Your pelvic floor exercises may be made more difficult by changing positions. It is best to begin your exercises lying down because you will be less affected by the downward pull of gravity. This position also encourages concentration and focus on isolating the proper muscle. Next progress to sitting, followed by standing, then walking, jumping, running, etc.

Exercises need to be progressed gradually in order to strengthen the muscle. Do not worry how long it takes, just listen to your body and keep challenging the muscle.

2. Increase the Length of Each Contraction

A second progression is increasing the time you hold each long hold contraction. You may begin holding a contraction for three seconds and resting for six seconds. When a three-second hold is easy to maintain, progress to a four-second hold (with an eight-second rest), then a five-second hold (with a ten-second rest), and so on. Increase your contraction to a ten-second hold. There is no need to increase your rest period greater than ten seconds since your endurance will be building during this time. If you are using the sample exercise program, then you will increase your five-second hold with a ten-second rest, to a six-second hold with a ten-second rest. Continue progressing toward a ten-second hold with a ten-second rest.

3. Increase the Number of Contractions

A third progression is increasing the number of repetitions in each set. If you have chosen to use the sample exercise program then you will begin with five repetitions of the long hold contractions and five quick contractions. When the fifth repetition feels as strong as the first repetition, then it is time to increase the number of repetitions. Increase from five to six repetitions, then to seven, and gradually to ten. For simplicity when counting, you may want to keep the number of long hold contractions and the number of quick contractions the same.

You will be working toward an exercise program of ten repetitions, holding each long hold contraction for ten seconds with a ten-second rest period, ten quick contractions and completing ten sets per day. At the beginning it is important not to over exercise your muscle. If you cannot feel the muscle tighten, stop and try again later. **Over-exercising the muscle is not beneficial.**

This may sound like a lot of exercise but really it is not. You will be doing ten sets per day and each set takes approximately one to two minutes to complete. This may be difficult to fit into your schedule when starting your exercise program as you need to take the extra time to lie down, double your rest period and focus on your contraction. This will become much easier as you progress and are able to incorporate your exercises into your daily activities. We will discuss this further in Chapter 14: Red Dot Program.

A chart has been included for you to keep track as you complete your exercises. Mark each of the ten sets as they are completed. Record the position the exercises were performed in;

L = Lying
S = Sitting
St = Standing
W = Walking

Sunday of Week 1 has been filled in as an example. Note that all exercises in your first week should be completed in a lying position.

Week 1	Sun.	Mon.	Tues.	Wed.	Thurs.	Fri.	Sat.
Position	L L L						
Long Hold	III IIII III						
Quick	III IIII III						

Week 2	Sun.	Mon.	Tues.	Wed.	Thurs.	Fri.	Sat.
Position							
Long Hold							
Quick							

Week 3	Sun.	Mon.	Tues.	Wed.	Thurs.	Fri.	Sat.
Position							
Long Hold							
Quick							

Week 4	Sun.	Mon.	Tues.	Wed.	Thurs.	Fri.	Sat.
Position							
Long Hold							
Quick							

Week 5	Sun.	Mon.	Tues.	Wed.	Thurs.	Fri.	Sat.
Position							
Long Hold							
Quick							

Week 6	Sun.	Mon.	Tues.	Wed.	Thurs.	Fri.	Sat.
Position							
Long Hold							
Quick							

Physiotherapist's Viewpoint…

As mentioned earlier, women with incontinence are eager to begin their home exercise programs. The first time we meet, women usually cannot wait to get home so that they can get started. They are excited to finally be able to do something about their incontinence and thrive on the idea that they may regain control over something so distressing in their lives.

The most frequent obstacle is not motivation, but rather, simply forgetting to do the exercises. Women have busy schedules, and it takes time to incorporate a new routine. Do not worry; this is a common problem. Keep working at the exercises, and eventually they will become a good and easy habit.

On occasion patients overdo their exercises. If they are given ten sets per day, they do fifty sets. These patients are motivated!

One woman mentioned that her pelvic floor had not had this much action since her honeymoon. Another woman was concerned that she was leaking more than ever and her muscles felt stiff and achy, especially her stomach. This all made sense since you cannot begin any exercise program at this level of difficulty. If you fatigue a muscle in the body, you will deplete its oxygen supply, and this may increase the risk of injury. If you continue exercising this muscle to its fatigue threshold, inflammation and micro-trauma may result. This is the cause of delayed onset muscle stiffness; the resultant soreness in muscles when beginning a new exercise program or sport. We have all felt this pain, and it resolves in a few days. If this happens to you, rest for two to three days and then resume your exercise regime, but at a slower pace.

For the pelvic floor muscle, you will want to avoid this experience since exhaustion of this muscle may lead to an increase in leakage, and you will be delayed in your exercise routine. In addition, as the correct muscle becomes exhausted, your accessory muscles (abdominals, gluteals and hip adductors) will start to do the work. Just like the patient whose stomach was sore, she did the exercises incorrectly just to get them done. **It is always better to do fewer exercises properly than more exercises using the wrong muscles**. Take your time. It took many years for your muscle to get to its present state of weakness, and it will take time to build it back up.

Key Points

• Pelvic floor muscle exercises are important to improve muscle strength and endurance, as well as to regain the urethral-closing reflex.

• Do your exercises in a quiet room so that you may focus and concentrate. Remember to breathe while exercising.

• Isolate and contract the pelvic floor muscle only, not your accessory muscles (abdominals, gluteals and hip adductors).

• When you start exercising, you will probably notice that the pelvic floor muscle will fatigue quickly. A good practice is to rest between each contraction for twice as long as the contraction itself. If the contraction was three seconds, then rest for six seconds before your next three-second contraction. Once you have progressed to a five-second hold with a ten-second rest, there is no need to further increase your ten-second rest period, since your muscle endurance will be improving.

- To fully exercise your pelvic floor muscle, you will need to perform long hold contractions as well as quick contractions. This will develop the two types of fibers within the muscle.

- Progress your exercises in three ways:

  1. Position changes
  2. Increasing the time held for your long hold contractions
  3. Increasing the number of repetitions of long hold and quick contractions

- Once you progress to ten repetitions of a ten-second long hold contraction there is no need to add more. To further challenge your muscle, see Chapter 21: Pelvic Floor Exercise Progression.

Did You Know?

Kegel exercises are named after gynecologist Dr. Arnold Kegel, who discovered the value of these pelvic floor exercises in the 1940's.

Chapter 13: Am I Doing It Right?

It is important to know what muscle you are exercising. Many women unknowingly use accessory muscles in place of the pelvic floor muscles. The incorrect muscles that are often substituted for the pelvic floor muscle are abdominals, gluteals and hip adductors. These muscles should be relaxed during pelvic floor exercises.

Many women erroneously think that doing a pelvic tilt is a pelvic floor contraction. With a posterior pelvic tilt, you roll your hips backward and flatten out the lower curve in your back. While this is a very good exercise, it will not strengthen your pelvic floor musculature. Remember, when you do your pelvic floor contraction properly, your body should not move.

The following are ways to test yourself to see if you are contracting the proper muscle:

While on the toilet, sit with your knees slightly apart and feet flat on the floor. Start your urine flow and then try to stop it. If you can easily stop the flow of urine, then you are using the proper muscle, the muscle you want to be exercising. If the urine flow is decreased or even somewhat deflected, this is still probably the correct muscle; it is just very weak and gives an ineffective contraction. **This activity is to be used only as a test of muscle strength and improvement, and should not be used as an exercise.**

Exercising during urination interrupts the coordination of messages being sent between the pelvic floor muscle and the urinary bladder. These muscles should not be contracted at the same time; they should work in an opposite fashion. As the bladder contracts the pelvic floor should relax, and vice versa. Over time, performing pelvic floor contractions while voiding (and your bladder is contracting to empty) can lead to problems with urgency.

Did You Know?

You should **not** be doing your pelvic floor exercises on the toilet.

Secondly, you may check to see if the proper muscle is being used by trying to stop the passage of gas from your anus. When you tighten your anus, you should feel the skin being pulled up and away from the chair you are sitting on. If your buttocks or thigh muscles move at all, then you are using the wrong muscles. Your body should not show any movement. The person sitting next to you should not be able to tell that you are exercising.

A third way to test if you are using the proper muscle is by physically assessing the muscle yourself. Wash your hands thoroughly or place a new disposable glove on your hand, and moisten the tip on your index finger with lubricating jelly or saliva (hand lotions may cause tissue irritation). Insert the tip of your index finger into your vagina about two to five centimeters (one to two inches). Now begin your pelvic floor muscle contractions around your finger. You should feel a tightening or pressure around your finger. Make sure that you are not tightening your abdominal or buttock muscles.

A fourth check is to look at what you are doing. Place a hand-held mirror between your legs. Try to view a tightening or movement of your perineum (the area between your legs) during the pelvic floor contraction.

If you are uncomfortable or unable to test yourself, or unsure if you are contracting the appropriate muscle, please see a qualified health care professional for assessment. Often if people do not see improvement in bladder control with pelvic floor exercises it is because they are not doing the exercises correctly. Many physiotherapists are now involved in continence therapy and seeking their advice may prevent disappointment and frustration if you are performing the exercises incorrectly.

Physiotherapist's Viewpoint...

A urologist once related a story about a patient who had been doing her exercises on the toilet. With each void she would try to start and stop the stream.

As this patient's muscle gained strength, she became very good at stopping her urine flow. Unfortunately, she became so good that she squirted urine back up into her bladder and triggered a kidney infection.

This is probably not a common occurrence but this story will stick in your mind. Never do your exercises on the toilet. It is acceptable to stop your urine flow on occasion to test your muscle for improved strength, or when you need to take a midstream urine sample (good luck). It is not good practice to routinely contract your pelvic floor muscle while your bladder muscle is contracting. When it is time to void, relax and urinate.

Key Points

- People often substitute accessory muscles when trying to do a pelvic floor contraction. Make sure that you are not using your abdominals (tummy muscles), gluteals (squeezing your buttocks) or hip adductor muscles (pressing your knees together).

- If in doubt, seek out a health care professional trained in pelvic floor muscle assessment to evaluate your exercises.

- Do not do your exercises while voiding.

Did You Know?

One study showed that when women received verbal instructions on how to do Kegel exercises, 51% performed them incorrectly and 25% used a technique that may actually increase incontinence symptoms.[13]

Chapter 14: Red Dot Program

Often women have difficulty getting into the routine of doing their daily exercises, and it can be overwhelming to commit to a lifelong exercise program. They are motivated, but their busy schedules may interfere and these new exercises can be easily forgotten.

Once endurance has developed, some women choose to get all their exercises done in the morning and know that their daily commitment has been completed. Others find that there is no time in the day to set aside for exercise. As time goes on it will be easier to complete your exercises, since, as endurance builds in this muscle, you will no longer have to separate your exercise program into three different times of the day. You may choose to do five sets of exercise in the morning and five sets at night, or all ten sets before your morning shower. If this works for you, then keep this routine. If you are still having difficulty getting them completed, then the following suggestions may be helpful.

Try to incorporate your exercises into your activities of daily living. Make a list of twenty activities that you do almost every day and then use these as cues to tighten up.

Incorporate Exercises into the Following Activities

- Brushing your teeth
- Riding in an elevator
- Standing up from sitting
- Sneezing
- Coughing
- Leaving a message on an answering machine
- Watching TV commercials
- Checking the time on your watch
- Stopping at a red light/stop sign
- Listening to the beat of a song
- Drinking water
- Stair climbing
- Shaving your legs
- Hand washing
- **After** you have completed voiding

For myself, I incorporate my pelvic floor exercises into other activities that I had trouble remembering to do. For example, I do my exercises while drinking water to increase my water consumption, and while flossing my teeth, to make my dentist happy!

In some cases, it is beneficial to add a visual stimulus to remind yourself to do your exercises and this is where the Red Dot Program can help. Many physiotherapists use this very simple technique as a reminder to patients to do their exercises. For some patients it is used to cue postural correction while other patients are reminded to do their neck stretches. Naturally, my patients use it as a trigger to tighten up. Just place red stickers on areas where you often look.

Places to Stick Red Dots

- Fridge door handle
- Car steering wheel
- Purse shoulder strap
- Watch wrist band
- Alarm clock
- TV remote
- Corner of your computer screen
- Telephone receiver
- Baby bottle warmer
- Microwave
- Toothbrush
- Answering machine
- Blow dryer
- Dental floss
- Water cooler
- Breast pump (providing you do not experience any interference with milk let-down when contracting your pelvic floor while breast-feeding).

Every time you see the Red Dot, do your exercises. Remember, after one to two weeks these dots will begin to blend into the background and you will no longer notice them. Use this time to establish a routine. If you require more time, simply replace the stickers with one of a different color so that they will stand out again. Whether you choose to incorporate your exercises into your daily activities with or without the use of red dots, remember to switch between your long hold contractions for strength and endurance, and your quick contractions to regain your urethral-closing reflex. In this way you will strengthen both types of fibers within the muscle.

Again, once your muscle endurance has built up, you may choose to complete all ten sets of your exercises first thing in the morning. For other people it will be easier to no longer count their exercises but instead incorporate them into their daily activities. Most people like to use a combination of both.

Physiotherapist's Viewpoint...

It is helpful to let your husband know why there are red stickers on the car steering wheel and the TV remote control. I have had patients report that they forgot to do their home exercise program because their husband removed the Red Dots, assuming that the kids had put the stickers everywhere. Have your husband use the Red Dots as a reminder to do some pelvic floor exercises too.

Other patients have had their kids relocate the stickers. One mom said it was a great idea that her eight-year-old kept sticking the red dots on his nose. Whenever she kissed her son, she remembered to do some exercises.

Key Points

- The biggest problem with a daily exercise program is remembering to do it. Combine your exercise with activities of daily living.

- Use the Red Dot approach as a reminder to do your exercises.

Did You Know?

Chocolate contains caffeine—sorry. Eat it in moderation (for further details see Chapter 15: Bladder Irritants).

Chapter 15: Bladder Irritants

Micturition, or voiding, is the act of emptying urine from the bladder. When sitting on the toilet, you relax your pelvic floor to begin this process of bladder emptying. This relaxation then triggers a reflex message to the brain. Next, the central nervous system will reply with a message to the bladder advising it to contract and empty.

As discussed in Chapter 4: The Nervous System, it is important that the pelvic floor muscle and the bladder muscle always work together but oppositely. During the filling stage the pelvic floor muscle should contract, while the bladder muscle relaxes. The reverse occurs during the emptying phase; the pelvic floor muscle and the urethral sphincters relax, and the bladder contracts to eliminate urine. This coordination of the pelvic floor and bladder muscles does not work in perfect combination for everyone. There are many factors that may cause disruption to this coordination. Bladder irritants frequently prevent pelvic floor and bladder muscles from working in unison.

Diet and lifestyle play a significant role in bladder continence. Certain foods and habits are irritating to the inner bladder lining and cause the bladder muscle to spasm in contraction at inappropriate times. This leads to the intense sensation of urgency to void. If left untreated this may develop into urge incontinence.

Following is a list of bladder irritants common to most women. It is best to remove bladder irritants from your diet one at a time over a period of two to three weeks. This will allow you to isolate the foods that are irritating to your bladder. If there is no decrease in symptoms during this period, then this particular food does not bother your bladder and it may be added back into your diet. If it is found to be an irritant you will want to avoid this food. Some bladder irritants affect one person very significantly while having no affect on others.

Acidic Fruits & Juices

Acidic fruits may exacerbate your incontinence symptoms. Orange, lemon, lime, grapefruit and pineapple fruits and juices are irritating to the bladder lining for many women.

Did You Know?

Juices like apple and grape are considered bladder-friendly whereas orange, grapefruit and pineapple can be irritating to the bladder. Cranberry juice is controversial. First, many people incorrectly assume that cranberry cocktail drinks are cranberry juice when there is only a small amount of actual cranberry juice in many of these drinks. Secondly, while some research indicates the benefits of cranberry juice in preventing and treating urinary tract infection, it can also be very irritating to your bladder lining and contribute to urgency symptoms. If your goal is to prevent bladder infections, cranberry pills can be very effective and do not tend to irritate the bladder.

Alcohol

Alcohol causes frequency of urination since it is a diuretic and increases urine output. Also, you may not react as quickly to the messages informing you of the need to void. Alcohol may impair coordination, balance and effective muscle contraction of the pelvic floor. It may take longer to get to the washroom since muscles may not be working optimally when under the influence of alcohol.

Did You Know?

Alcohol is a diuretic and therefore it removes water from your tissues and other storage areas and sends it to your kidneys. This causes you to excrete more water than you have consumed.

Artificial Sweeteners

Artificial sweeteners can be found in diet drinks and many diet foods. People with diabetes often rely heavily on adding artificial sweeteners to their food as an alternative to sugar. Unfortunately, like caffeine, artificial sweeteners can be a cause of bladder irritation for people experiencing urgency. Some foods, like diet yogurt, contain artificial sweetener in some brands, while other brands of low fat yogurts do not. You need to read the food and drink labels.

Caffeine

Caffeine is a stimulant and a diuretic and can be found in coffee, tea, chocolate, cola and certain medicines. Caffeine is irritating to almost all individuals, and if you are suffering with urgency or urge incontinence, it should be eliminated from your diet completely or consumed sparingly. It is important to remove caffeine from your diet gradually to prevent caffeine-withdrawal headaches.

Did You Know?

Caffeine consumption leads to urgency and frequency.

Carbonation

Carbonated beverages such as sodas and sparkling waters often irritate the bladder lining. Any fluid with bubbles may be aggravating to the tissue and lead to urgency symptoms.

Constipation

A full bowel places pressure directly on the urinary bladder, causing an increased pressure within the bladder that may push urine outward. This pressure may also stretch the bladder wall and trigger a false message of bladder fullness.

Straining during a bowel movement produces a downward pressure that over-stretches the pelvic floor muscle. Make sure that your diet is rich in high fiber foods, such as whole grain cereals and breads, and fruits and vegetables. This will decrease your risk of constipation. If you suffer from chronic constipation, try to eat a minimum of five fruits and vegetables each day (according to Canada's Food Guide that suggests five to ten servings per day) and increase your non-caffeinated fluids, especially water.

Fluid & Water Restriction

Try to drink six to eight (250 milliliter/eight-ounce) glasses of fluid, with the majority being water, each day. Concentrated urine is a very significant irritant to the bladder lining. If you notice that your urine has an odor, or is dark yellow or orange, increase your fluid consumption. You should not be able to smell your urine as you void; if you can, you need to drink more water.

Remember that many fruits and vegetables, such as watermelon and lettuce consist mainly of water and therefore can be included in your total daily fluid intake. As well, foods that are liquid at room temperature, such as ice cream, also qualify as liquid. It is best to drink more fluids throughout the day and less toward bedtime.

Did You Know?

Your normal daily fluid intake should be between 1500 to 2000 milliliters (forty-eight to sixty-four ounces). Sugared fluids (such as fruit drinks, soft drinks and Kool-Aid) and caffeinated beverages (such as coffee and colas), are not to be included due to their dehydrating effect.

Medications

Certain cough medicines, over-the-counter drugs, and prescription medications can affect continence. Read labels and ask your pharmacist for suggestions on substitutions. The following drugs may cause temporary urinary incontinence or increase existing incontinence: antihistamines, anti-psychotics, antispasmodics, anti-Parkinson agents, calcium channel blockers, diuretics, sleeping pills or sedatives, decongestants, and antidepressants. The effects of medication on bladder control was discussed in greater detail in Chapter 9: Factors Related to Incontinence.

Red Food Dye

Red food dye may also irritate the bladder lining and is found in many sandwich meats and wieners, as well as some baked goods and candies (such as red licorice).

Smoking

Nicotine itself irritates the lining of the bladder and therefore may produce urgency. A chronic smokers-cough puts continuous stress and pressure on the pelvic floor musculature causing micro-trauma (small tearing) and weakness to the region leaving it at risk of injury.

Spicy Foods

Spicy foods such as Mexican, Thai, Cajun, and Indian dishes may irritate your bladder, as well as your bowels. This can contribute to urinary and fecal incontinence. Also, when there is bowel irritation, diarrhea and constipation may result, putting stress and strain on your pelvic floor. If this occurs frequently over long periods of time, it may produce dysfunction in this region.

Sugar

Sugared foods and beverages promote dehydration and therefore may contribute to concentrated urine (which is a bladder irritant). Sugar does not need to be eliminated from your diet, but avoid consuming high quantities of sugary treats and beverages.

Physiotherapist's Viewpoint...

When first studying female incontinence many years ago, I was still drinking several cups of caffeinated coffee and consuming many diet colas each day. Thankfully, this was before having my beautiful babies and my pelvic floor muscle and bladder still tolerated my bad diet. I would not be so lucky now.

At an incontinence seminar I attended, a physician gave a presentation regarding the effects of diet on bladder control. He stressed that patients wanting to regain continence must eliminate coffee, artificial sweetener, alcohol and smoking from their lives. I remember sitting there trying to hide my coffee and diet cola, and thinking that if patients were asked to do exercises for life and give up their coffee, they may never return for treatment. I decided to concentrate on strengthening exercises first, and worry about diet once patients developed a good exercise routine.

It did not take long to realize that this decision was not in the best interest of the patient. I usually waited until patients had been doing their exercises for a few weeks and then casually mentioned that coffee may be playing a role in their leakage and urgency.

Many patients then chose to eliminate caffeine from their diets. On more than a handful of occasions, women returning for their follow-up appointment had given up coffee and as a result were dry. At that point I gave up diet cola, cut back on coffee and was forced to admit that diet was a very critical factor in bladder control for many women, and it should never be overlooked.

Similar experiences occurred with artificial sweeteners. There is often a pattern noted with patients who have been diagnosed with diabetes. Once diabetics switch their sugar intake to artificial sweeteners, they frequently begin to experience urinary incontinence. This is **not** to say that diabetic women should choose sugar over artificial sweeteners. Their blood sugar level is a far greater medical concern than incontinence. This is simply a reminder that artificial sweeteners should be used sparingly. People with diabetes may want to discuss this with their physician.

Not every woman is affected this dramatically by diet. Many patients have told me that they get away with one cup of coffee and remain dry, but with two cups the problems begin. Other patients report that they cannot tolerate a single cup of coffee, others not a sip.

From these experiences I have learned that it is not my place to hold back potentially helpful information. Today's women seek all the advice and information they can get. When they are empowered with this information, they are able to make informed decisions that fit their lifestyle.

They may choose to decrease coffee consumption rather than eliminate it. I ask patients to think twice before having a cup. Do they really want one? Then they should have it and enjoy. If it is simply a social beverage, choose a glass of water instead. Remember that these may be big changes, so expectations need to be realistic. This should not be viewed as starting a new diet but rather improving the existing diet.

Even if diet is found to be a major factor in your urinary leakage, your exercises are still important. You will want to work on every area that you have control over to see the best results. If your muscle is strong, you may just get away with a cup of coffee and a piece of chocolate cake—once in a while.

Key Points

- Many diet and lifestyle choices may have negative effects on bladder control. Some people will be greatly affected by one food while that same food has no affect on another person.

- Bladder irritating foods may cause the bladder to involuntarily contract when it should be in a relaxed state, thus producing a feeling of intense urgency.

- The irritants that affect bladder continence most dramatically are caffeine, artificial sweetener, alcohol, smoking, and concentrated urine.

Did You Know?

Often wearing a sanitary pad gives women the license-to-leak. Try to remove this security blanket as soon as you can. Also, wearing tampons may provide extra support and therefore temporarily decrease your symptoms. However, it is not a good idea to have a tampon inserted at all times. This is only a crutch to the problem and may lead to tissue irritation and possible infection.

Some women experience sensitivities to certain brands of sanitary pads. It is a good idea to experiment with the many types available.

Chapter 16: Bladder Diary

To gain insight on the functioning of your bladder it is often beneficial to track what goes into and out of your body. Keeping a bladder diary will allow you to notice trends or problems (that you may not otherwise be aware of). A Bladder Diary has been included in this chapter so that you may log your bladder habits. You will also find a sample diary as an example. You may list many variables on a single chart. The more information you collect, the easier it will be to improve your bladder habits.

Food & Beverage Input

Mark all fluid intake and note the type and amount of each beverage you drink. Logging your food intake will also identify items that are irritating to your bladder lining. If a food becomes a liquid at room temperature, like ice cream, then it should be included in your 1500 to 2000 milliliters (forty-eight to sixty-four ounces) per day fluid count. Some fruits and vegetables, like watermelon and lettuce, have a high water content and need to be taken into consideration when you are deciding if your bladder actually requires emptying, or if it is a false message of urgency.

Bladder & Bowel Output

Now monitor your urine output throughout the day. Use a measuring cup for accuracy, or purchase a urine collector from a pharmacy. This device is often called a urine or toilet hat and it simply sits under the toilet seat and catches the urine as you void. The urine hat has markings to allow easy output measurements.

There will be many occasions that prevent actual measuring of urine output. Most women do not want to carry a measuring cup in their purse when they leave the house or go to work. For these situations, simply count the number of seconds you urinate and compare these to previous measurements when you have both counted and measured. This may not be a precise figure but it will give you a good estimate. A rule of thumb is that you urinate approximately one ounce for every second you count.

You will also need to record your bowel movements. If you are seeing a physiotherapist, you may be asked to note your bowel movements, presence of constipation or diarrhea, and to quantify the amount of pushing and straining needed to empty your bowels.

Bladder Irritants

Take note if you have consumed any bladder irritating foods or beverages. See Chapter 15: Bladder Irritants, for a listing of foods most commonly aggravating to women; however, there may be other diet items specifically upsetting to your bladder.

Urine Leakage & Urgency

Keep track of any urinary leakage episodes or strong urges. Mark the size of the leakage (small, medium or large) as well as the activity you were doing during the leak, for example aerobics or sneezing. Also mention whether or not you were able to delay your urge (see Chapter 18: Urgency & Urge Delay Techniques).

Voiding Dysfunction

Write down any problems you have had with initiating your urine flow, intermittent urination (urine flow stops and starts), or if you felt you could not fully empty your bladder.

Keep track of this diary for three to seven days. This may be a difficult and time consuming task; however, the more information you gather the easier it is to locate problems. Just do your best, even one day of tracking can be helpful. Now carefully review your diary

- Did your output correspond to your input?
- How many times during the day and night do you urinate?
- Does leakage occur after eating a certain food?
- Was urgency related to certain diet factors or activities?
- Were you able to successfully delay the urge?

Included in this chapter is a sample bladder diary followed by a blank bladder diary for you to photocopy and track your input and output. Good luck.

Sample Bladder Diary

	Tuesday	Wednesday	Thursday	Friday
6:00 am	Awoke with urge Small leak Void 200mL	Awoke with urge Small leak Void 300mL		Awoke with urge Void 100mL
7:00 am	Awoke with urge Small leak Void 100mL	Aerobics Large leak Void 200mL	Awoke to alarm Void 350mL	Aerobics Large leak Void dribble
8:00 am	2 Caff. Coffee White toast Grapefruit	2 Caff. Coffee Cereal/milk Grapefruit	2 Caff. Coffee Pancakes Void 200mL	2 Caff. Coffee White toast Grapefruit
9:00 am	Muffin 1 Caff. Tea Void 300mL	Small leak with lifting		Void 6 seconds
10:00 am	Leak with cough Void 4 seconds	1 Caff. Coffee Muffin	1 Caff. Coffee Granola bar Void 12 seconds	1 Caff. Coffee Muffin
11:00 am	Diet cola Apple	Void 15 seconds		
Noon	Taco Rice Diet cola Void 15 seconds	Void 8 seconds Lemonade Chili Salad	Void 10 seconds Hot Dog Fries Diet cola	Void 21 seconds Pizza Diet cola Void 7 seconds
1:00 pm	1 Caff. Coffee	Diet cola		Void 7 seconds

2:00 pm	Bowel movement with straining Void dribble	Void 15 seconds	1 Caff. Coffee Void 8 seconds	1 Caff. Coffee Chocolate bar Void 9 seconds
4:00 pm	1 Caff. Coffee Chocolate bar	Strong urge Small leak Void 8 seconds		Small leak while walking
5:00 pm	Void 8 seconds before leaving work	Void 4 seconds before leaving work	Void 12 seconds before leaving work	Void 8 seconds before leaking work
6:00 pm	Strong urge Small leak on arriving home Void 50mL	Urge at home Void 8 seconds	Urgency with medium leak Void 6 seconds	Mild urge Void 4 seconds
7:00 pm	Spaghetti Salad Wine	Meat Loaf Carrots Wine	Soup & Salad 1 Caff. Coffee Chocolate ice cream	Hamburger Fries Chocolate cake Beer
8:00 pm	1 Caff. Coffee Chocolate Cake	Popcorn Diet cola	Void 300mL	Void 15 seconds
9:00 pm	Void 350mL	Small leak with laugh	Diet cola Potato chips	Nacho/sauce Beer
10:00 pm	1 glass water Diuretic pill	1 glass water Diuretic pill	1 glass water Diuretic pill	Void 25mL

11:00 pm	Void 300mL Go to bed	Void 450mL Go to bed	Void 350mL Go to bed	Small leak standing up
Midnight	Awoke with urge Void 100mL		Awoke with urge Void 250mL	1 glass water Diuretic pill
1:00 am		Awoke to void 150mL		Void 350mL Go to bed
2:00 am				
3:00 am			Awoke to void 150mL	Woke with urge Small leak Void 5 seconds
4:00 am			Awoke to void 150mL	
5:00 am				

Did You Know?

The average amount a person voids ranges from 250 to 500 milliliters (eight to sixteen ounces).

Suggestions for this Diary

- Reduce or eliminate caffeinated coffee consumption (gradually taper down to avoid withdrawal headaches).
- Remove diet drinks and artificial sweeteners from diet.
- Increase fluid consumption, especially water, to six to eight glasses per day.
- Begin urge delay techniques and gradually increase the time span between daily voids to decrease frequency symptoms. Special attention should be made to decrease voiding and urge during the night (see Chapter 18: Urgency & Urge Delay Techniques).
- If taking a prescribed diuretic, talk to your doctor to see if you can take your medication in the morning instead of just before going to bed. This may decrease the need to void during the night.
- Fully relax the pelvic floor muscle when voiding to completely empty bladder. Watch toileting posture (see Chapter 20: Toileting Posture).
- Begin a pelvic floor muscle-strengthening program immediately (see Chapter 12: Proper Pelvic Floor Exercises).
- Increase intake of bran, fiber, fruits and vegetables, since one bowel movement in four days may indicate problems with constipation, and straining is harmful to the pelvic floor.
- Decrease consumption of spicy foods, chocolate and alcohol.
- Switch morning grapefruit to an apple or banana.

Key Points

- It is important to track what goes in and out of your bladder.

- When you have several days marked, study your habits to note problem areas and then create a plan to improve them.

	Day 1	Day 2	Day 3	Day 4	Day 5
6:00 am					
7:00 am					
8:00 am					
9:00 am					
10:00 am					
11:00 am					
Noon					
1:00 pm					
2:00 pm					

3:00 pm					
4:00 pm					
5:00 pm					
6:00 pm					
7:00 pm					
8:00 pm					
9:00 pm					
10:00 pm					
11:00 pm					

Midnight					
1:00 am					
2:00 am					
3:00 am					
4:00 am					
5:00 am					

Did You Know?

It is very important to maintain your fluid intake, especially water. It is equally important to not become over-hydrated. 3500 milliliters (100 to 120 ounces) of daily fluid is too much liquid for most women, as this may re-set their thirst receptors making them feel thirsty more quickly. Aim for 1500 to 2000 milliliters (forty-eight to sixty-four ounces) of fluid each day.

Chapter 17: Urinary Frequency

Frequency is a common symptom associated with bladder dysfunction. Women often experience symptoms of frequency and urge before they actually begin to leak urine; however, these symptoms initially go unnoticed and as they increase, they are usually ignored. Therefore, urinary frequency and urgency are most often left untreated. Frequency is the need to void more than five to nine times in a day, and more than once during the night. With aging comes an increased need to void during the night and it is acceptable for the elderly to void greater than one time per night. If you need to void more often than every two and a half to four hours, then you are experiencing frequency. When left untreated, frequency may progress to urinary incontinence.

Use your bladder diary to track your voiding schedule. Should you find that you are using the washroom more frequently than every two and a half to four hours or more than five to nine times a day, gradually work on increasing the time intervals between voids. If you have pain when trying to delay voiding, you should see your physician.

Frequent bladder emptying will result in shrinkage of bladder capacity. It will now take less volume to trigger the stretch receptors in the walls of the bladder to send a message to the brain reporting the need to void. This becomes a cycle of increasing frequency and decreasing the bladder capacity. The volume of urine being emptied per void will decrease. You must break this cycle to regain normal bladder size by eliminating this dysfunctional voiding behavior. It will take time for your bladder to enlarge to its proper size again; be patient and look for gradual improvements.

If you are voiding every hour for example, then postpone your urination to every one and a half hours. When this becomes easy, try to extend to two hours, and so on, up to the acceptable range of every two and a half to four hours.

Remember to use common sense. If you just drank two glasses of water and ate watermelon, then your bladder is full and will need to be emptied, no matter when your last void took place. Should you urinate less than five times per day, check your bladder diary to ensure an adequate fluid intake. Urinating should take at least eight to ten seconds. If your void only lasts for four or five seconds, you did not need to empty your bladder.

Physiotherapist's Viewpoint...

I was once at a conference where, without being aware of it, we (the participants) were monitored as to our liquid consumption and washroom use. It was really embarrassing when this group (who should know better) were discovered to be going to the washroom every time we had a break in our course schedule, even when it had only been one hour since our last break.

This was a good learning experience for me. It had become a habit that at lunch and breaks I would quickly go to the washroom to avoid having to interrupt an interesting lecture. It is easy to pick up bad habits of voiding 'just-in-case', or every time you leave the house. Most of us learned to do this as children: run to the washroom before you get into the car even if you had no feeling of needing to void.

After having my second baby I realized that I had created another bad habit, I started to go to the washroom whenever I woke up at night to nurse. While you are breast-feeding, you will probably consume a lot of water and it may be necessary to empty your bladder during the night. However under normal circumstances, if you are not breast-feeding, you should not need to void more than once at night. When my daughter finally started to sleep through the night, I was still waking up to go to the washroom. Again I was trapped in a bad habit, and I should have known better.

Once you realize your mistake, it is easy to correct with urge delay techniques and calming thoughts. These will be discussed in the following two chapters. The critical component is recognizing that there is a problem.

Key Points

- Urinary frequency is the need to void more often than five to nine times during the day and more than one time at night.

- Frequency is often left untreated and may progress to urinary incontinence.

Did You Know?

Do not void 'just-in-case' since this may lead to frequency. You do not always need to urinate just because you are leaving the house. Think about how long it has been since your last void and how much fluid you have consumed before you automatically go to the washroom.

Notes

Chapter 18: Urgency & Urge Delay Techniques

Urgency

Urgency is the strong urge with an immediate need to void. This is also often referred to as an overactive bladder. As mentioned in Chapter 15: Bladder Irritants, urge may be related to bladder irritating foods and lifestyle. Urgency does not necessarily include urine leakage. However, incontinence may follow the urge if you are unable to reach the washroom in time. Stress incontinence usually produces small amounts of leakage, or dribbling, whereas urge incontinence is often associated with large leaks, or flooding. Stress incontinence is usually predictable in occurrence, while urge incontinence can be completely unpredictable.

For whatever reason, be it bladder irritating foods and beverages such as coffee, or concentrated urine annoying to the bladder lining, when you experience urgency your bladder muscle has begun to contract when it should be relaxed. This voiding dysfunction needs to be addressed.

Many women complain that the only time they experience urgency is when they are at home or pulling into their driveway. This is such a common phenomenon that it is known as the key-in-the-door syndrome. When approaching the security of their home, some women are overcome with urgency and may lose bladder control, even when they have just gone to the washroom. For some women the urge is triggered by passing the washrooms in a mall or rest areas on the highway. Washing dishes or simply the sound of running water may also be difficult.

Often our central nervous system plays a significant role in urgency and therefore a large amount of concentration and effort will be required to calm the bladder muscle and delay urgency. For many women, the incredible urge that sends them dashing to the washroom only to void a pathetically small amount, is a learned behavior. This pattern must be unlearned. Most of these women will know the location of every clean washroom in town and, finding it difficult to pass one by, will instead stop at each one to void 'just-in-case'.

Urge Delay

Now that you have begun your home exercise program and are able to locate and contract your pelvic floor muscle, it is time to use this ability to calm urge. Initially, your goal will be to postpone the need to void just long enough to reach the washroom. Gradually you will increase this delay time to eliminate any problems with frequency.

When a strong urge develops it is important to remain as calm and relaxed as possible. Try to contract your pelvic floor muscle slowly and gently, this will promote relaxation of the bladder muscle (it is this bladder muscle that is responsible for the strong desire to void). This is a reflex that we want to restore. When the bladder muscle and pelvic floor muscle are working properly and in coordination, one muscle should be relaxed while the other is contracted. When we feel a strong urge, this is the bladder beginning to contract when it should be relaxed. By contracting the pelvic floor musculature we are attempting to reinstate a reflex that sends a message to the bladder instructing it to relax. For a more detailed explanation of how this reflex loop functions, see Chapter 4: The Nervous System.

To further dampen the urge, as you contract your pelvic floor, try to relax your mind. Anxiety and panic feed the urge sensation. Immediately running to the washroom will usually lead to incontinence along the way. When your feet hit the ground you will put further pressure on your bladder and interrupt the contraction of your pelvic floor muscle as it attempts to close the urethral sphincters.

You may want to sit down or lean on a nearby counter or wall while contracting your muscle and calming your mind. This will encourage relaxation and decrease the abdominal contraction that may be contributing to the pressure on your bladder.

Now that you are contracting your pelvic floor and trying to relax, remind yourself to breathe. Holding your breath will increase anxiety while depriving your muscles of oxygen at a time when they need it the most. Once you have completed four or five contractions, try to relax and assess how your bladder muscle is doing. Has the need to void passed completely? If so, continue going about your day as if the urge had never happened. Try to wait to void until you think your bladder actually needs to be emptied, which is either after sufficient fluid intake or two and a half to four hours since your last void.

If the urge has decreased but not resolved, repeat the process and then reassess. If the urge is still very strong, then slowly and calmly walk to the washroom and void. Repeat this urge delay technique with every urge.

This urge delay should be progressively increased. If you are able to dampen the urge by even a small amount, this may allow you the confidence to walk, rather than run, to the washroom. Once this gets easier, try to delay for one full minute. Add one minute every time you feel that you are able to increase your delay time. It may take several weeks and a considerable amount of concentration to calm the urge for a full five minutes. When this is no longer difficult, try for ten minutes, then fifteen minutes, and so on until you are able to completely calm the urge and are voiding only at appropriate times.

Trying to calm urge is extremely difficult, but it is of the utmost importance. If you are suffering with urgency symptoms, then your bladder is taking control over you. It is essential that you stop this cycle and control your bladder symptoms. If the urgency/frequency cycle is allowed to continue, it will become progressively worse and eventually control your daily activities. Most people benefit from any form of distraction. Involve yourself in your work or in any activity that takes your mind off your strong bladder urge. Hum a tune, count backwards, read or turn on the television or radio.

Another option is perineal pressure. When an urge begins, apply pressure to your perineum (the space between your legs) and physically lift your pelvic floor to prevent leakage. You may use your hand, a rolled up towel, or even the corner of a table to do the job that your weakened pelvic floor musculature is not yet able to do. As your muscle strength increases, these techniques will no longer be needed.

It is perfectly acceptable to clench your accessory muscles while trying to delay an urge. You may need them. Many women cross their legs and use their hip adductors (inner thigh muscles) to hold the urine in. Use whatever means you have available. It is only when you are exercising your pelvic floor that you must isolate it from your accessory muscles.

Physiotherapist's Viewpoint...

The following are a few clinical examples of how an overactive bladder can impact one's life.

Urgency

A patient once told me an interesting story of why she finally told her doctor about her incontinence. This forty-five-year-old grandmother was teaching her granddaughter how to use the toilet. The potty training process had been slow, but on this particular day they were making progress. As her granddaughter sat on the toilet she excitedly shouted for joy "I'm peeing Gramma!" and they both cheered. As the grandmother listened for the dribbling noise (to tell if it was really working this time) one of her many daily urges kicked in. It was so intense that she pulled the little girl and her potty seat off the toilet as she pulled down her own pants to void a few drops. When she looked up, her granddaughter was crying as pee dripped down her legs.

What had begun as an exciting accomplishment quickly became a very upsetting and embarrassing experience, leaving both of them in tears.

This lady made an appointment with her doctor and sought help. Six months later she was able to delay her urge by fifteen to twenty minutes. At the last sleepover at her house, even when she was experiencing an urge to urinate, she was able to wait for her three grandchildren to pee first, before she did.

It took a lot of hard work for this determined woman to build up to this level. Trying to relax urge is often the most difficult challenge for patients trying to normalize their bladder habits, but it is extremely important. If she had done nothing about her problem, her urges would have occurred more frequently and probably also increased in intensity. You have to break this cycle and stop feeding the urge and perpetuating the pattern. If this lady had not conquered her bladder dysfunction, in all likelihood she would have eventually experienced more embarrassing situations and gradually may have spent less time with her grandchildren and more time alone at home.

Please never let bladder problems restrict the activities you want to participate in. Should you encounter bladder symptoms, do not keep this to yourself. There are many people who want to help, talk to your doctor or seek out a physiotherapist who has a special interest in incontinence. Urgency may occur for other reasons such as bladder outlet obstruction (or prostate enlargement in men), and it is therefore necessary to seek medical help from your physician.

Key-In-The-Door-Syndrome

I recall a humorous story of one patient's experience with the key-in-the-door syndrome. On her daily return home from work she noticed that familiar pressure on her bladder as she turned onto her street. This urge increased as she passed each of her neighbors' houses. She was already in the habit of voiding at work before her fifteen minute drive home, since urgency was such a common occurrence for her. By the time she pulled up on her driveway she was clenching her legs together, as well as her teeth. As she got out of her car, she stepped in a pothole and then felt a flood. She had lost complete control of her bladder with the sudden jolt of her stumble. Furious and embarrassed, she ran into the house and yelled at her husband to fix the pothole. Well, needless to say the driveway was quickly repaired but we all know that the real problem was not resolved.

This woman did very well with treatment and driving home is no longer torture, even when I suggested she stop going to the washroom 'just-in-case' before leaving work. Both she and her very understanding husband are happy and proud of her accomplishment.

Pediatric Urinary Incontinence

Our clinic has had the pleasure of treating children as well as adults with bladder and bowel dysfunction. This book is focused on female urinary incontinence but since heredity does increase the risk of incontinence, I thought some mothers might find this interesting.

We often see a similar key-in-the-door syndrome in children, while on the bus ride home from school. As they near their home they often experience urinary leakage. This problem is not quite the same with children as with adults and it is therefore treated differently. I ask my adult patients to avoid using the washroom before leaving the office unless it has been two and a half to four hours since their last void. However, I ask children to please go to the washroom before they leave school. I have seen many children who void only two times in a twenty-four hour period. Children have smaller bladders and should void more frequently than adults (they just rarely have the time).

Key Points

- Urge delay techniques are very effective in calming your bladder and decreasing the feeling of urgency:

  Step 1. Sit down or lean on a nearby wall or counter.

  Step 2. Contract your pelvic floor to trigger the reflex leading to relaxation of the bladder muscle. Some people prefer to hold one long contraction while others choose several shorter contractions. Trust your instincts.

  Step 3. Try to remain calm, anxiety will increase the urgency.

  Step 4. Remember to breathe.

  Step 5. Reassess the urge. Is it less intense or gone altogether? If it is gone, just return to your day as if it had not happened. If it improved but is still present, repeat steps 1 through 5.

- Delaying urgency will not be easy and may take several months before you are able to sufficiently delay the urge.

- Many women find that distraction and perineal pressure are helpful. Use the corner of a table, your hand or a rolled up towel to lift your perineum. You may want to cross your legs for extra support. Distract yourself any way you can.

Did You Know?

People experiencing incontinence should not wear tight clothes that press on their bladder and are difficult to remove quickly.

Chapter 19: Relaxation Techniques

The nervous system has a significant effect on the urination process. It is important to learn to relax your mind and hence the nervous system, and your bladder, as we did with the urge delay techniques. This will instill a calming influence over your nervous system and mind and body as a whole. The following techniques can be used to diminish anxiety and mental stress that may over-stimulate nerves, producing symptoms of urgency.

Visualization

When trying to relax your mind and bladder, it is often helpful to picture the bladder muscle itself in a spasm. Try to view this tight, angry muscle letting go, expanding and relaxing. Now picture your whole body becoming relaxed as anxiety and tension float away. Visualization is a powerful aid.

Breathing

Remember your breathing. Diaphragmatic breathing is simply the process of breathing in deeply so that air is moved down to your diaphragm. You do not want to be an 'upper-chest-breather' since rapid and shallow breaths will limit the movement of air and it will enter only the upper portions of your lungs. If you are breathing correctly, you should see a rise and fall low in your abdomen and not in your chest. Deep air entry is necessary to increase the amount of oxygen your muscles receive, making them healthier and to improve their function.

Concentrate on calming thoughts as you slowly breathe in through your nose and out through your mouth. Exhalation (breathing out) should be longer than inhalation (breathing in). Breathe in through your nose for a count of three seconds, and out through your mouth for five to six seconds. It is often helpful to purse your lips as the air exits you mouth. This slow and controlled breathing pattern works to further decrease tension and anxiousness.

Relaxation

Some women also benefit from relaxation techniques such as audiotapes of birds or ocean waves (other women complain that the sound of rushing ocean water is the last thing they would want to hear), candles, soft lighting and music. Use whatever audio or visual techniques you find relaxing.

Warm Thoughts

It is often beneficial to think of warm situations, such as lying on a beach in Hawaii, where you feel relaxed and calm. This can actually increase your body temperature and direct blood flow to certain areas of your body. Imagine blood and warmth being circulated to your bladder and pelvic floor. Increased blood flow causes an increase in body temperature and oxygen to your muscles. With more oxygen reaching your muscles, the bladder and pelvic floor will function better. Women with urinary incontinence often complain of having cold hands and feet. Visualize your hands holding a hot cup of cocoa or coffee and your feet soaking in a hot bubble bath. By doing this you can increase the blood flow to your hands and feet, warming these areas and encouraging better circulation throughout your body.

Positive Thinking

Positive thinking can also be very beneficial. Repeat to yourself:
"I will not leak, and I will not run to the washroom." or
"I will decrease this urge; I will not let my bladder run my life."
If you tend to leak urine when you are in a stressful situation or
a strong urge comes on, remind yourself that you are in charge
of your bladder. It is not the other way around. Tell yourself
that you deserve to be dry. While doing your pelvic floor
contractions, visualize the bladder relaxing and think of your
body as being warm and calm.

Between trying to delay urge and using the relaxation
techniques, you may find yourself confused as to when to do
what. Try all of these ideas and see what works for you. Most
people combine a few tricks to customize their own protocol.
For example, when you feel an urge beginning, you may lean on
the counter and lift your perineum (the area between your legs)
with your hand. Now contract your pelvic floor as you begin
diaphragmatic breathing. Try to distract and relax your mind with
calm, warm thoughts. Reassure yourself that you will be dry, you
deserve to be dry, and that you are stronger than your bladder.
You may need to adjust your techniques from one urge to the
next. Encourage yourself by looking for small improvements
so that you may see benefit in continuing the techniques and
prevent frustration and disappointment.

Physiotherapist's Viewpoint...

One patient reported urinary leakage when she was at the office
and under a sudden mental stress. She became nervous when her
boss entered her office to ask a question. As her anxiety increased,
she began to leak urine. Naturally, she then became even more
flustered and felt her face turn red and hot. She found that she was
unable to answer with the professional and appropriate response
that quickly came to mind once her boss left her office.

Stress affects people very dramatically. Mental strain can produce tension on the pelvic floor muscle, leaving the contraction weak and uncoordinated and therefore unable to properly close the urethral sphincters. For treatment we worked on strengthening her pelvic floor muscle, removed some major bladder irritants from her diet (especially coffee at work), and developed an urge delay program. What made the most dramatic improvement was teaching her to remain calm, using a variety of techniques. After four months, this young woman rarely experienced incontinence. I met this patient at the grocery store a few years later and she cheerfully told me that her boss had been fired.

Key Points

- Relaxing and calming the nervous system is critical in regaining bladder control. Use whatever techniques you find helpful.

- The central nervous system and its complex reflexes play a large role in bladder function. Never underestimate the effect of mental strain and stress on your body.

Did You Know?

Approximately 20 million people in North America suffer from paruresis (par-yū-rē'sis), or shy bladder syndrome. This is a disorder where people have difficulty or are unable to urinate in public washrooms or places where others may hear them.[14]

Chapter 20: Toileting Posture

As children, many of us were never told that there are right and wrong ways to urinate. Who would believe that as an adult someone would correct us on something that we have done independently for decades, something so simple and so personal. I am afraid that many of us are unaware that what we do mindlessly several times every day may qualify as poor habits that can lead to voiding dysfunction. The following are descriptions of common errors made during urination.

Pushing

A harmful mistake that many women make is pushing during voiding. Urination should always be a **passive** event. To actively push out urine requires abdominal muscle contraction, and when we use our abdominals we tend to tighten up our pelvic floor muscle. This makes it more difficult to eliminate the bladder contents and it becomes necessary to force the urine out. Remember, the pelvic floor should be relaxed and the urethral sphincters fully opened. When voiding, the bladder muscle will contract and with the assistance of gravity, urine drains. Aim for a slow and steady, rather than a forced, stream.

Breathing

Another mistake is forgetting to breathe. Breathing promotes relaxation while ensuring good oxygen delivery. When children are having voiding problems, we ask them to blow on a pinwheel to encourage breathing or else to count aloud the number of seconds they peed. This will discourage pushing and breath holding, while making them more aware and involved in their voiding process.

Valsalva Maneuver

The Valsalva maneuver is the inappropriate technique of holding your breath and pushing to empty your bladder and bowels. It is so commonly done that it actually has a name. It is very important for us to stop bearing down on our pelvic floor in such a manner. Any woman with a prolapsed uterus will have learned the hard way that if they Valsalva, it often feels like they may deliver their uterus. Do not wait until you are at this stage to correct your toileting habits. Try to change now and decrease the stresses on your pelvic floor. This is also information that we should pass on to our children when potty training.

Voiding on an Empty Bladder

When asked if we void less then eight to ten seconds, how many of us would know the answer? Most adults never give this a thought. Well, I am sure you will notice now. You will also notice if the woman in the next public stall only urinated for three or four seconds. Make sure that when you empty your bladder you really need to and that it is not the bad habit of 'just-in-case' voiding, or an urgency/frequency syndrome.

Hovering

Another error when voiding is hovering. Women have a tendency to crouch or hover over the toilet seat, especially in public washrooms. This is a bad habit because quadricep and abdominal muscle contraction is necessary to maintain this posture and, as we already know, reflexively we will experience contraction of the pelvic floor. This again leads us into the poor voiding pattern of forcing urine through our pelvic floor musculature and urethral-closing sphincters. When you are in a public washroom, you may want to use toilet paper or a paper cover to line the seat. This may alleviate some of your discomfort regarding sanitation and allow you to sit and fully relax your muscles to begin the passive event of voiding.

Posture

When sitting on the toilet make sure that you are in a comfortable position. If you are of short stature you may need to support your feet with a small stool or phone book to bring your hips and knees to the same level as the toilet seat. This may also be helpful if using an elevated toilet seat for other medical reasons. Do not squeeze your thighs together. Sit up straight, relax your pelvic floor muscle and legs and allow urination to begin.

If you have difficulty starting the urine stream, your pelvic floor musculature may be in spasm. It is important to learn to relax the pelvic floor muscle. If the urine flow starts and stops, we refer to this as staccato peeing and it is another dysfunctional voiding pattern. It is important to fully relax the pelvic floor muscle to allow the urine to be eliminated. If you are unable to correct this pattern please seek treatment with a physician or physiotherapist qualified in the treatment of urinary dysfunction.

Some women feel that they have not fully emptied their bladder when urine flow has stopped. In this situation they should shift their weight from side to side and lean forward. Relax the pelvic floor and more urine may be excreted. Some women might even have to stand up and then sit back down to empty the last amount of urine. This may tilt the bladder into a position that promotes drainage. During menstruation, if you wear a tampon it needs to be removed before voiding. The tampon serves as a type of pessary and may prevent complete emptying of the bladder. Pessaries will be discussed in Chapter 24: Available Treatment Options. To fully empty their bladder, men may need to sit during urination instead of standing, since standing also tends to promote a forced urine stream.

Remember, after you have finished urinating or defecating, **tighten up** your pelvic floor muscle as you stand-up. This will complete the job by giving a good signal to the bladder to stop contracting and relax, and to close off the urethral sphincters. Now the bladder-filling phase can begin again.

Physiotherapist's Viewpoint...

One sweet woman reported urinary leakage one to two minutes after voiding. She would usually be washing her hands when she felt that all too familiar trickle. For treatment, we naturally began addressing her diet and initiating a home muscle-strengthening program. We reviewed her positioning on the toilet and found that her legs barely reached the floor. She was asked to slide a telephone book under her feet and then work on techniques to fully relax her pelvic floor muscle. As we reviewed her history, it revealed that she often hovered over public toilet seats and then needed to push hard to force the urine out. Years of this behavior, compounded by being rushed in the washroom by her young children, produced muscle tension in her pelvic floor.

Proper postural correction combined with Computerized EMG Biofeedback training (see Chapter 25: Physiotherapy for the Pelvic Floor), taught this patient to relax her pelvic floor when voiding, allowing her to empty her bladder more completely. She was also asked to take more time in the washroom (I realize this is next to impossible when she often had her one-year-old child on her lap and her three-year-old banging on the door). Once she finished voiding she readjusted her positioning and then relaxed for an additional thirty to sixty seconds. During this time she visualized her pelvic floor relaxing and was able to urinate a few more drops.

Since cold running water had been a trigger to her leakage, we also added techniques to calm her nervous system (see Chapter 19: Relaxation Techniques) and asked her to use warm water for hand washing. This woman was dry in less than one month.

Key Points

- Voiding is a passive event; never push.

- Never hover over the toilet seat. Sit down and relax your pelvic floor muscle.

- If you are having difficulty learning how to properly relax your pelvic floor, seek the help of a qualified physiotherapist or incontinence specialist trained in Computerized EMG Biofeedback.

Did You Know?

Pelvic floor weakness and laxity can lead to poor anal positioning. This may cause constipation, difficulty with emptying your bowels, decreased control with holding back gas, and urinary and fecal incontinence. To make fecal elimination easier, insert two fingers vaginally and gently push backward toward the anus. This support will better position the anus and therefore prevent unnecessary straining.

Chapter 21: Pelvic Floor Exercise Progression

O nce your daily pelvic floor exercise program becomes easy, you will want to challenge yourself further. You are ready to progress if you can do the following easily:

- Locate your pelvic floor musculature at will.
- Feel that your pelvic floor musculature gives a good, strong contraction with no accessory muscle use.
- Contract your pelvic floor musculature for a seven to ten second hold.
- Contract your pelvic floor musculature for seven to ten repetitions without muscle fatigue (both long hold and quick contractions).
- Contract your pelvic floor musculature while performing other activities of daily living such as talking, reading or watching television.

It may take you anywhere from one month to one year to develop your pelvic floor muscle to the point that you no longer have difficulty recruiting this muscle contraction. Do not be concerned with the length of time it takes to progress to this stage of muscle strength, endurance and overall awareness of your pelvic floor. When you feel ready, try the following exercises to help achieve a higher level of control over your pelvic floor:

- The Wave
- The Elevator
- The Ball Lift

The Wave

Physiotherapists practicing in the field of Women's Health often prescribe a pelvic floor exercise known as The Wave. For this exercise you will begin contracting from back to front. The first time you try this exercise you should assume the original exercise position of lying on your back with two pillows, or a stool, under your knees. Make sure that you choose a quiet room with no distractions so that you may concentrate on your exercise. Do not forget to breathe.

Begin contraction of your pelvic floor muscle at the posterior aspect, or muscle fibers in the back around your anus, just like when you do not want to pass gas. Now progress your contraction in a forward direction, from anus to vagina to urethral opening, until you can feel a tightening near your pubic bone, at the front of your pelvis. You should now be contracting the whole muscle. Relax, and try it again. This helps to build awareness and control over different segments of the muscle. Most women find it easier to contract near the anal region and more difficult to control the fibers in front by the urethra. Keep concentrating on the anterior, or front, fibers and eventually these will be much easier to contract.

The Elevator

Another good exercise used by many physiotherapists is The Elevator. For this exercise, visualize your pelvic floor muscle as being on the main or ground floor during its normal resting state. Now, bring your pelvic floor muscle to the second floor with a very minimal contraction. Increase it to the third floor or a mid-level contraction and then finally bring it to the fourth floor, that being a maximal contraction of your pelvic floor. Slowly reverse the process. Go down to the third floor, second floor, and then the main floor. It is much harder to control going down the floors than going up.

Next, try to bring your pelvic floor muscle to the basement. Be careful not to bear down on the muscle but instead gently try to open the urethra, vagina and anus. You need to be able to open your pelvic floor for normal bowel and bladder emptying.

Now, come up from the basement to the main floor, that is, the normal resting tone for this muscle. Never leave your muscle in the basement or on the fourth floor. Always bring it back to its normal resting state when you have completed your exercises (or after voiding). Your normal resting tone is a low level muscle contraction that you are unaware of. This low level muscle contraction is necessary for preventing bladder leakage.

The Elevator

Note: Main Floor is the Pelvic Floor Resting Level.

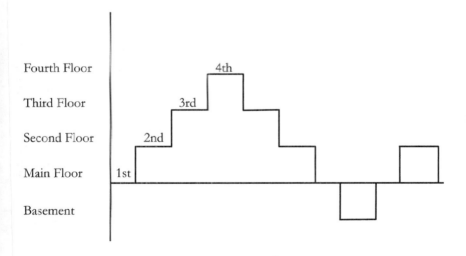

The Ball Lift

Strength is only one important element in gaining control of your bladder. Another is muscle control, being able to have the muscle contract as much or as little as you want it to. A wonderful technique to work on this is imagining that you are lifting a ball with your pelvic floor muscle. First visualize lifting a ping-pong ball, then a golf ball, and finally a tennis ball. Start in a sitting position and then progress to standing and eventually squatting. You should notice your strength change when accommodating to different weights and sizes. This exercise is an excellent way of teaching your pelvic floor to open-up. This is the same technique you would use to move from the main floor to the basement in the elevator exercise.

You may want to do a few repetitions of these exercises every few days. They may be tricky to begin with, however, after much practice you will be surprised at the improvement in control you will gain over this muscle. Keep working on these, they will get easier.

Physiotherapist's Viewpoint...

A physical therapist once told a story about an elderly woman who leaked urine whenever she bent down to pick up her cat. The therapist showed the patient where her pelvic floor muscle was located, how to contract it, and explained how it worked to close off the urethra when you increase your intra-abdominal pressure, as with lifting. This lady very quickly learned to contract her pelvic floor muscle properly and her therapist instructed her to tighten up as she picked up her cat. When she returned for her follow-up appointment, she had been dry all week. Further treatment was not indicated since the patient had full bladder control once she knew how to accommodate for the loss of her urethral-closing reflex. Naturally, she was reminded to continue her home strengthening program for maintenance.

Key Points

- After exercising or voiding, tighten up your pelvic floor so that it regains its standard level of closure. This ability to maintain a low level of contraction in a resting state makes this muscle quite unique from other musculo-skeletal muscles.

- Once you have mastered your pelvic floor exercises, try The Wave, The Elevator and The Ball Lift exercises. These exercises will increase your coordination and control over the pelvic floor muscle.

Did You Know?

To stretch the pelvic floor you simply have to squat. It has been said that women who live in countries where they work in the fields in a squat position all day, never experience bladder incontinence. A healthy muscle will know how to stretch and contract.

Notes

Chapter 22: Accessory Muscle Exercises

If you are having difficulty doing your pelvic floor exercises, or if you just do not have enough time in the day to get them done, then it is probably not wise to start additional exercises. However, as you feel your pelvic floor muscle increasing in strength, and you have found a routine for your daily exercises that fits into your lifestyle, it is time to start a strengthening program for your whole body.

You will want to strengthen your stomach, lower back and upper leg muscles so that they may better assist the pelvic floor in supporting your bladder and other pelvic organs. Strengthening muscles surrounding your pelvis will take some of the stress off of your pelvic floor muscle, as well as increasing blood circulation to the pelvic region.

It is also important to begin the habit of contracting your pelvic floor before using your abdominal muscles. This will strengthen your urethral-closing reflex and counteract the downward pressure placed on the pelvic floor. Whenever the intra-abdominal pressure increases, the downward pressure can lead to an over-stretching of the pelvic floor musculature and therefore weakening of the muscle. The following exercises will promote this habit of tightening your pelvic floor before you contract your stomach muscles. This behavior is essential and should be incorporated in all daily activities.

These exercises are to be completed in addition to your daily pelvic floor exercises, and should be done three times per week. If you have a busy week and are unable to do your exercises, these are the exercises to decrease or omit, not your daily pelvic floor exercises. Remember to breathe while exercising.

The following are five exercises to achieve accessory muscle strengthening. Exercises 1, 2 and 4 have progressions to continuously challenge your muscle.

Exercise 1

Lie on your back with your knees bent. Your feet should be flat on the floor and slightly spread apart.

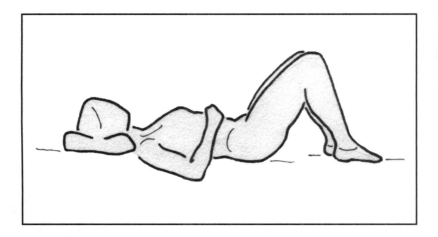

Step A

Begin by contracting your pelvic floor muscle. While holding this muscle tight, contract your abdominal muscle by pulling your belly button inward toward your spine and upward toward your head. You should feel your stomach harden. Now count ten seconds. You may want to count aloud to encourage breathing while you exercise. Now relax your abdominals, and finally, relax your pelvic floor. Your pelvic floor should be the first muscle to contract and the last to relax.

Complete this exercise as many times as you are able to do it properly. You will want to work up to ten repetitions. It is always better to do two exercises correctly than ten exercises poorly.

If you find that you cannot hold your pelvic floor contraction for a count of ten, you may want to adjust your exercise to a five-second hold. Once you are able to correctly complete a ten-second exercise and repeat this ten times, you are ready to progress this exercise to step B.

Step B

The next step is to add a pelvic tilt. Begin by contracting your pelvic floor muscle. While holding it tight, contract your abdominal muscle by pulling your belly button inward and upward. You should feel your stomach harden. Now add in a posterior pelvic tilt by flattening your lower back toward the floor and removing any arch in your lower back. Hold this contraction for a count of ten. Relax your low back, then relax your abdominals and finally relax your pelvic floor. Work up to a ten-second contraction that you are able to repeat ten times. When this is achieved, progress to step C.

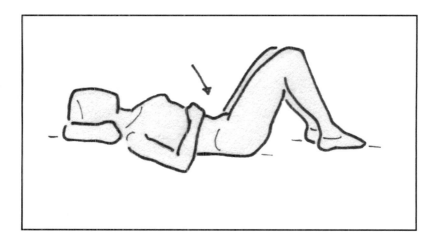

Step C

Step C will add a partial sit-up. Begin by contracting your pelvic floor muscle. While holding it tight, contract your abdominal muscle by pulling your belly button inward and upward. You should feel your stomach harden. Now raise your shoulders and head off the ground approximately six inches, and reach for your knees. Hold for ten seconds, and then lower your head and shoulders back to the ground. Relax your stomach and finally your pelvic floor. Work up to a ten-second contraction for ten repetitions.

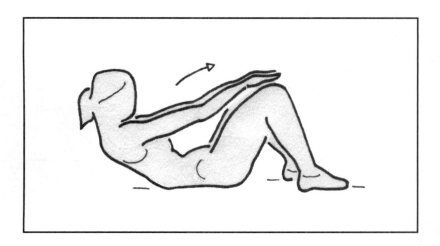

Exercise 2

Now that you have worked on strengthening your pelvic floor, abdominal and low back muscles, we need to address the gluteal muscles (glutes).

Step A

While sitting on a hard chair or stool, begin contracting your pelvic floor muscle. Maintain this contraction as you squeeze your gluteal, or buttock, muscles together. You should feel your body lift up and off the hard seat. Hold this for a count of ten. Relax your glutes and then your pelvic floor. Work up to a ten-second contraction for ten repetitions. When this is achieved, progress to step B.

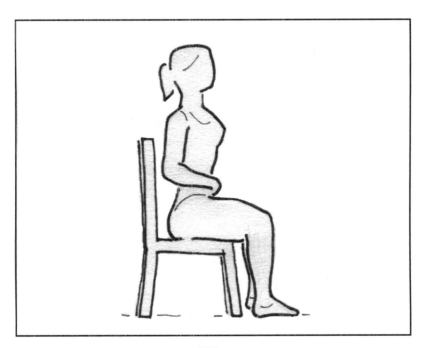

Step B

Step B will add in a bridge position. This progression will incorporate your pelvic floor, abdominal, low back and gluteal muscles. Lie on your back with your knees and hips bent. Place your feet flat on the floor and slightly separated.

Begin by contracting your pelvic floor. Pull your belly button inward and upward, and flatten your back toward the floor. Next squeeze your buttocks together and raise your bum off of the floor into a bridge position. Make sure that you are fully tightening your pelvic floor, abdominal and gluteal muscles while maintaining a posterior pelvic tilt.

Hold this position for a count of ten. Next, bring your bum down to the floor and relax your buttocks, and stomach. Finally, you may relax your pelvic floor. Work up to a ten-second exercise, repeated ten times.

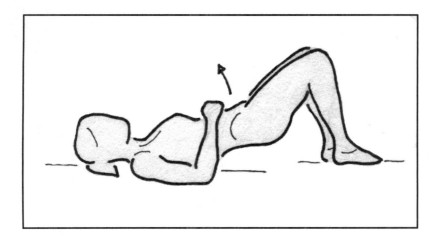

Exercise 3

Next you will need to strengthen the muscles controlling your hips. Lie on your back with your hips and knees bent. Place your feet flat on the floor and slightly separated. There are two parts to this exercise and they will contract different hip muscles. These are not progressions, and therefore Parts A and B should be completed.

Part A

For this exercise, you will need a four to eight-inch ball, or a pillow folded in half, placed between your knees. Begin by contracting your pelvic floor and then squeeze your knees together into the ball or pillow. Hold for ten seconds. Relax your legs and then your pelvic floor. Work up to a ten-second contraction with ten repetitions.

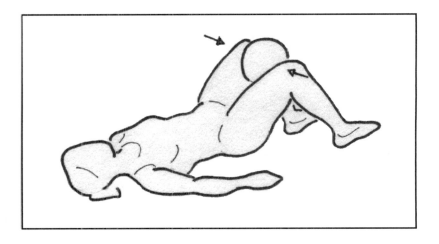

Part B

For this exercise you will need some rubber banding or an old pair of pantyhose. Tie your thighs together with the banding. Keep the band close to your knees. Begin by contracting your pelvic floor. Now pull your knees apart against the resistance of the band. Hold for ten seconds. Relax your legs and then your pelvic floor. Work up to a ten-second contraction with ten repetitions.

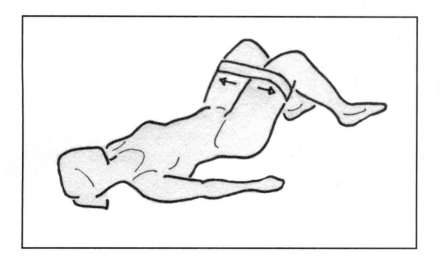

Exercise 4

This exercise will focus on the every day activities that cause a rapid increase in intra-abdominal pressure, while maintaining a pelvic floor contraction. Exercise 4 is important for reinstating your urethral-closing reflex, and may be done in sitting or standing.

Step A

Contract your pelvic floor and cough once or twice. Now relax your pelvic floor. When you are able to do this without leaking, gradually increase the strength of your cough and work up to ten coughs at a time. If it is difficult to tell whether or not you have leaked urine during your cough, you may want to place a folded tissue into your underwear so that it will be easier to note any wetness. This will also allow you to monitor the decrease in the amount of leakage, as the wet circle becomes smaller in size.

Step B

Repeat Step A substituting a fake sneeze for the cough. Again work up to ten sneezes while holding your pelvic floor contraction, gradually increasing the intensity of the sneeze.

Step C

Begin sitting on a chair or stool. Contract your pelvic floor and then stand up. Relax your pelvic floor and assess for leakage. Work up to repeating this ten times.

Step D

This again uses the format of Steps A and B but with the activity of blowing your nose. Contract your pelvic floor muscle while you blow your nose. You may also work up to ten repetitions for this exercise but more importantly, use this as a way to work into a habit. Just like bringing your hand to your face when you cough or sneeze, you should contract your pelvic floor every time you cough, sneeze, rise from a chair or blow your nose. Also, remember to make this a habit whenever you lift an object.

Exercise 5

For this final exercise you will need to be creative. Think of any activity that has caused you to leak urine in the past. You may want to write out a list. The best way to strengthen a muscle is to perform a specific activity over and over. Create your own exercise and think of ways to develop a progression when you achieve bladder control during this activity. The following are some exercises that may give you ideas when customizing an appropriate exercise for yourself. Maintain a pelvic floor contraction while:

- Stair climbing. Start with one stair and progress the number of stairs as you are able to maintain bladder control until you are able to ascend and descend a complete flight of stairs.
- Standing on one leg. When this no longer causes leakage, lift up on your toes or gently bounce.
- Jumping on the spot. Begin jumping with both feet, then progress to one foot.
- Running on the spot.
- Swinging your golf club.
- Pretending to throw a curling rock.
- Cross country skiing.
- Skateboarding.
- Skipping.

So far, all of the exercises in this book are specific to the pelvic floor itself and the accessory muscles that assist the pelvic floor in supporting the pelvic organs. The rest of your body will also require some form of exercise. Any increase in body weight will put extra strain on your urinary bladder and pelvic floor musculature and therefore increase your risk of incontinence. General exercise may take the form of walking, running, swimming, sports, or any activity that you find enjoyable and will promote weight loss, circulation and overall general fitness.

Physiotherapist's Viewpoint...

In physiotherapy school, a professor asked us to develop an exercise program for a teenager who had been in a car accident and would spend the rest of his life in a wheelchair. Our assignment was to create an exercise program to prepare his body for this physical challenge.

My group came up with an elaborate program using specialized strengthening equipment to focus on various muscle groups. We were on the wrong track. A much more effective program would have been to let him use his own wheelchair.

It was an important lesson to learn. Muscles will develop best when doing the function we want to reproduce. It is beneficial to strengthen the supporting and assisting muscles as well, but always recreate the activity with which you are having difficulty.

I once treated a long distance runner who was having trouble with urinary leakage. With strengthening exercises she was able to remain dry, provided she did not come across any potholes or obstacles that required sudden lateral movement. She also was greatly affected by cold and damp weather.

Initially, we had her running indoors on a treadmill to remove all lateral disturbances and weather changes. Once she regained bladder control at this level, we added in one challenge at a time. She did a lot of pelvic floor exercises standing with her legs spread wide apart. We then added jumping to her routine and, finally, running a course requiring lateral movement over obstacles.

To deal with the weather, we worked on calming her central nervous system (see Chapter 19: Relaxation Techniques).

She worked hard for a full year before she felt confident enough not to wear a pad when running outdoors. She continuously challenged herself and taught me never to settle for improvement but always to push for resolution.

Key Points

- It is important to strengthen the rest of your body as well as your pelvic floor. Strengthening your accessory muscles adds support to your bladder.

- Exercise increases the blood circulation and therefore improves the health of the muscles and tissue.

- Always tighten your pelvic floor before superimposing an increase in intra-abdominal pressure onto it. Remember to contract your pelvic floor during activities that previously caused urinary leakage.

Did You Know?

Many competitive female athletes suffer from urinary incontinence. Exercising the rest of your body is not good enough; you must strengthen your pelvic floor muscle as well.

Notes

Chapter 23: Signs of Regaining Bladder Control

Once you have formed a sound exercise routine and are faithfully doing your ten sets of pelvic floor exercises every day, you will be anxiously awaiting the results of your hard work. You must realize that initially these improvements may be small. You need to take notice of these minor changes because otherwise you may become frustrated and give up on your exercises. It will take time for muscle strength and endurance to build, and control over your bladder to return. The problems did not arise overnight and rarely will the correction.

Initial changes range from very small, to complete resolution of urine leakage and all bladder symptoms. When improvement is noted immediately, it will be too soon to be attributed to gains in muscle strength, but rather it is probably the result of isolating a dietary factor that is especially irritating to your bladder. Sometimes the removal of caffeine or artificial sweeteners can have this dramatic effect. As well, improvement within the first few days of exercise may be related to your new ability to locate your pelvic floor muscle, so that you remember to tighten up before increasing your intra-abdominal pressure. This can also bring about dramatic improvement of incontinence very quickly for some women, as it did for the woman who leaked when she lifted her cat.

It is more common to see small improvements initially, and more notable increases in control approximately six to eight weeks into your exercise program. By this time you should feel that your exercises are becoming easier, and that you are able to hold the contraction longer.

After several months of exercise, the diameter of individual muscle fibers will enlarge and your muscle will be significantly stronger. With both strength and endurance increasing, your muscle will be able to contribute better closure to the urethral sphincters.

While you anxiously await development of pelvic floor muscle strength, remember to correct any poor voiding behaviors that may be contributing to your incontinence (such as voiding hourly, or pushing with urination). These changes may also produce early improvements. When you have been exercising for six weeks, it is often helpful to complete a second bladder diary to compare with your initial diary. This will provide you with objective numbers to contrast. Photocopy the chart found in Chapter 16: Bladder Diary.

Improvements To Look For

- The feeling of greater control over your bladder.
- A decrease in the number of incontinent episodes.
- A decrease in the amount of leakage during an episode.
- A decrease in the size of pads or number of pads used.
- A decrease in daytime or nighttime frequency.
- A decrease in the number of urge sensations.
- A decrease in the intensity of the urge.
- An increase in the time you are able to delay urge.
- An increase in muscle strength.
- An increase in muscle endurance.
- A decrease in accessory muscle use when exercising.
- Normalization in voiding behaviors: proper toileting postures and schedules.
- Resumption of activities previously avoided because of incontinence.
- An increase in confidence and self-esteem.

Should you note even small changes such as the ability to delay a strong urge for five minutes, this is significant and needs to be recognized. Think back to a time when you would have been thrilled to have an extra five minutes to make it to the washroom during a strong urge. It is important to see what a big step this is. It is natural to want immediate resolution of the problem, but it rarely works that way. Control takes time and hard work.

Why Continue Your Exercises?

If you are completely dry at six weeks, do not stop your exercises. First, **the muscle will weaken quickly if neglected, and symptoms usually return.** Secondly, your muscle has the potential of greater increase in strength and endurance if you continue exercising. This excess strength may serve as your safety zone if you decide to have a glass of wine on a special evening, or if you catch a cold with a bad cough in the future. **Do not stop exercising** when you have full control. You may not need to do as many exercises if you just want to maintain this level, but you will almost always regress if you stop exercising completely.

If you have not noted significant improvement in bladder control within two to three months of beginning your exercise program, you should seek assessment from your physician or a qualified continence health professional such as a physiotherapist. There are many options to explore in deciding what treatment is most appropriate to your health and lifestyle (see Chapter 24: Available Treatment Options, for further details).

Physiotherapist's Viewpoint...

For most women, after two or three months of their exercise routine, the increase in bladder control is usually unmistakable. By this time patients have often progressed from multiple daily leaks, to only one or two leaks each week.

Review your initial bladder diary to see the number of leakage episodes you had been experiencing. Often women who were leaking several times each day, and then improve to a single daily leak, undervalue this achievement since they are still incontinent. To remain motivated you must note this as a significant change, even though you have not yet attained the level of control that you want.

In the initial three to six weeks it is especially important to be aware of the small changes. When patients do not see the benefits, they may become frustrated, and give up on their exercises. Please do not stop! It may take time, but strength and endurance of a muscle are often slow to build. Just compare this muscle to all other muscles in the body that require time and energy to get them into shape.

Patients at both ends of the continuum of severity in symptoms may have difficulty noticing initial improvements. I ask patients with mild symptoms, who may only leak when they have a cough, to try to force several coughs. Count how many coughs it took to bring on a leak. Now use this number for future comparison. Be creative in finding ways to analyze your progress.

For one patient with extreme symptoms, who estimated leaking a few hundred times in a day, improvement was difficult to notice because she simply could not count the number of leakage episodes each day to assess. She also did not want to weigh her incontinence pads to accurately measure the amount of urine leakage.

She tried to count the number of pads used but this was also difficult since she was unsure how full they were. The sign she was looking for came when her husband asked why the grocery bills were so cheap the last few weeks. She realized that she was not buying nearly as many costly pads. This was the encouragement she needed to motivate herself to continue her exercise program.

On her last appointment at the clinic she was down to seven to ten small leaks per week. This patient confessed that she had not believed that she would ever improve and was thrilled with her achievement.

Whenever I meet a patient who makes me feel slightly overwhelmed by the severity of the symptoms, I just remember this patient and how great her improvement was. She is an inspiration.

Key Points

- It is important to notice small improvements so that you gain confidence and enthusiasm with your exercises rather than becoming frustrated and quit.

- It took a long time for the problem to build up, and it will take time to regain control.

Did You Know?

In 1996, more than $1.5 billion was spent on adult diapers. A person with incontinence typically spends $1000.00 to $3000.00 on absorbent products each year. It is also estimated that urinary incontinence accounts for 30% of all sanitary napkins sold. [15]

Chapter 24: Available Treatment Options

Aproper home exercise program and change in diet is all that is needed for most women to improve bladder control. However, if you are diligent with your exercises and there has been no improvement after two to three months, it is time to look at the treatment options available to you. If you have not seen your physician regarding your bladder symptoms, then you should do so now. When no improvement has been experienced it is often due to incorrect exercise procedure. When there is any doubt about locating and contracting your pelvic floor, and Chapter 13: Am I Doing It Right? did not alleviate your concerns, then it is time to see a professional. Physiotherapists with post-graduate training in Pelvic Floor Muscle Dysfunction would be appropriate for assessment of this muscle and bladder re-training treatment if necessary.

There are also options to discuss with your physician. Your doctor will be able to advise you on current medications and surgical techniques that may be appropriate for you. Some physicians offer pessaries to aid in support and bladder control. A pessary is an internal orthotic device worn to support the bladder or uterus. Pessaries come in all shapes and sizes. They are usually made of silicone, and easy to fold and insert into your vagina. Once in place, the pessary will spring back to its original shape and when fitted properly, you should not feel the pessary inside your body. Some women choose to remove the pessary daily for cleaning, while other women, often elderly, may choose to leave the pessary in place and return every three months to have their physician remove and clean it. Pessaries can be very effective and an excellent option when surgery is not appropriate.

Your physician should always be seen to rule out any underlying medical condition that may be causing incontinence, such as urinary tract infection. Further testing may be indicated, such as urodynamic bladder function assessments. Bladder testing will be discussed in Chapter 27: Bladder Function Testing.

In medicine there is rarely a universal remedy for any diagnosis, and that is why a team approach is often the most appropriate plan for treatment. It is important to seek out information on all available treatment options so that you may decide what is best for you. Some women find benefits from one form of treatment while other women do not. The following chapters will expand on these procedures.

Key Points

- If you have not seen any improvement after two to three months of faithful pelvic floor exercising, it is time to review your medical treatment options.

- If you have not already done so, see your doctor to discuss your bladder symptoms and to prepare your treatment plan.

Did You Know?

Many female pelvic pain disorders have a pelvic floor muscle component. When a muscle cannot fully relax it may be extremely painful. Think of how excruciating a cramp in your calf muscle can be, and imagine this in your perineum. It is just as important to be able to relax your pelvic floor muscle as it is to contract it.

Chapter 25: Physiotherapy for the Pelvic Floor

Physiotherapists (Physical Therapists in the USA) are trained health care professionals who treat dysfunction of the human body, usually injuries to the musculo-skeletal system. Some physiotherapists have a special interest in the area of Women's Health and choose to obtain post-graduate education to assess and treat the pelvic floor musculature.

Physiotherapists can offer conservative non-surgical treatment to help restore pelvic floor muscle strength and bladder control, or treatment can be used as an adjunct to pharmaceutical and surgical options. Education to correctly perform appropriate pelvic floor muscle exercise is an essential component in strengthening these muscles. Pelvic floor muscle retraining may include Computerized EMG (Electromyography) Biofeedback or Neuromuscular Electrical Nerve Stimulation Therapy. These treatment techniques help patients locate and contract the proper muscles while improving muscle strength. A certified physiotherapist may also offer acupuncture therapy to help with bladder control. Vaginal weights or cones may be used to further challenge and strengthen the pelvic floor musculature.

If you are not confident that you are performing the pelvic floor exercises properly, or if you have not achieved control over your bladder after two to three months of faithful exercise, you may choose to seek the help of a qualified physiotherapist for assessment.

Your physiotherapy visit should involve an extensive medical history documentation and physical assessment. You will receive education regarding topics such as:

- Proper Bladder and Pelvic Floor Function
- Bladder Diary
- Diet and Lifestyle Modification
- Urgency and Urge Delay Techniques
- Proper Toileting Postures and Schedules
- Bladder Retraining

Your therapist will customize a home exercise program for muscle strengthening. In addition, you may benefit from other treatment modalities to assist you in locating and better contracting the correct muscles. Your physiotherapist may offer programs such as:

- Computerized EMG Biofeedback Training
- Neuromuscular Electrical Nerve Stimulation/Electical Stimulation
- Acupuncture (in Canada)
- Vaginal Cones and Weights

Many physicians are choosing these conservative forms of treatment as an option for their patients either to prevent the necessity of surgical intervention, or as an adjunct to strengthen the pelvic floor musculature pre and post surgery.

Did You Know?

A study was completed in 1987 to document the effect education and pelvic floor strengthening exercises had on women with stress incontinence. The results: 100% of these women showed significant reduction in the number of incontinence episodes they experienced and 32% of these women were cured.[16]

Computerized EMG Biofeedback Training

Computerized EMG Biofeedback is used to measure the electrical activity within a muscle and transmit this information into a format that allows us to observe and objectify this movement. A second biofeedback channel reports any accessory muscle recruitment, bringing attention to improper muscle contraction. When the patient is able to visualize this, it can improve the awareness of the location of the muscle, as well as increase one's control over the muscle. When this is achieved, the next step is learning to contract and relax this muscle at will.

Did You Know?

Of the several types of urinary incontinence, stress, urge and mixed account for over 90% of all UI (urinary incontinence). Pelvic muscle weakness is usually prevalent with these three types of UI and these patients would be appropriate for EMG Biofeedback therapy.[17]

Studies on the various applications of biofeedback combined with behavioral treatment report a range of 54-87% improvement in incontinence across various patient groups using different biofeedback and behavioral procedures.[18]

Neuromuscular Electrical Nerve Stimulation

Neuromuscular Electrical Nerve Stimulation (NMES), also known as electric stimulation, can be used as a means of improving the ability to contract the pelvic floor muscle. This then allows the patient to continue their home exercises to increase the strength and endurance of the muscle. This modality excites the nerve, triggering contraction of the muscle. This type of therapy works very well for patients who may have difficulty contracting this muscle on their own, usually when it is very weak or injured. It is important to note that the use of a machine is temporary; it is a form of treatment and not an excuse to ignore your own exercise program. Physiotherapists always promote independence by using the benefits of this modality to bring the strength of the muscle to a level that your own exercises can be effectively performed. Machines cannot exceed what a healthy muscle can achieve.

Acupuncture

Acupuncture may be offered as an adjunct to standard physiotherapy treatment. The purpose of this modality is to regain a balance in the function of the nervous system. This treatment may be used for symptoms of urinary urgency, urge and stress incontinence and pelvic pain.

Vaginal Cones and Weights

Vaginal cones or weights may be used to challenge and further strengthen your pelvic floor musculature. They usually come in kits with the cones and weights ranging from less than one ounce to several ounces, to allow a graduated progression.

You simply insert a weight or cone into your vagina, just like you would a tampon, and then contract your muscles to prevent the cone from falling out. These can be used while you go about your regular daily activities in the privacy of your home. Some women have even tried to keep the cone inside their vagina while vacuuming. Cones and weights can be beneficial for muscle coordination problems. Pelvic floor cones and weights should not be used if you have a problem with chronic infections, if you are pregnant, within six weeks of having delivered a baby or undergone pelvic surgery, if you have an IUD in place, or during menstruation.

Physiotherapy Assessment

Physiotherapy assessment will identify contractility, strength, endurance, tone and symmetry of your pelvic floor musculature, as well as reflexes, skin sensation, pelvic pain, vaginal size and skin irritation or rash. There are many indications for physiotherapy assessment and treatment of the pelvic floor. Most commonly, patients present with one or more of the following:

- Urgency
- Urinary frequency
- Dysfunctional voiding patterns
- Urinary incontinence
- Fecal incontinence
- Pelvic organ prolapse
- Pelvic pain
- Pelvic floor muscle spasm
- Difficulty locating and contracting the pelvic floor muscle
- Questions regarding a pelvic floor home exercise program

As more women become aware of the physiotherapy treatment offered for Pelvic Floor Dysfunction, many see a physiotherapist for education in preventing loss of bladder control. More and more women want a good pelvic floor exercise program. Women are becoming more aware of the importance of this muscle and are unwilling to allow it to decrease in function.

Your physiotherapy assessment will be quite thorough and you will be asked questions you may never have given thought to. During an assessment, be prepared to answer questions regarding your symptoms. For example:

- When did the incontinence begin?
- How frequently does the leakage occur?
- What aggravates the problem?
- How many pads do you fill per day?
- Does anything decrease the amount of leakage or frequency of incontinent episodes?
- How many times per day do you void? Per night?
- Do you experience urgency?
- Do you have difficulty starting to void?
- Is the flow strong or weak? Does it start and stop?
- Do you dribble when you stand up?
- Do you have pain when you void?
- Can you feel when your bladder needs to be emptied?
- What color is your urine? Can you smell your urine?
- Have you ever found blood in your urine?
- Do you have back pain or pelvic pain?
- Do you feel heaviness or a falling out sensation in your perineum?
- Do you have trouble achieving sexual orgasm?
- Do you have trouble emptying your bowels or difficulty with constipation?

Did You Know?

If one parent suffered with nocturnal enuresis (bed-wetting) as a child, there is a 44% chance that their child will have problems as well. If both parents were bed-wetters, chances increase to 77%.[19]

Physiotherapist's Viewpoint...

Physiotherapy for Pelvic Floor Dysfunction may be appropriate for women with varying goals. Some women are simply seeking education and a proper home exercise program. This may require one or two appointments. For women whose pelvic floor muscle is extremely weak, or they are unable to locate this muscle without using their accessory muscles, a full treatment program may be indicated. Physiotherapy treatment varies from clinic to clinic but will often consist of two to three appointments per week for six to eight weeks. Treatment includes use of any of the modalities previously discussed depending on needs and symptoms.

A physician's referral may be required for physiotherapy treatment. This is often to satisfy a patient's insurance requirements. More importantly, the referral ensures that a medical health screening to rule out infection and any underlying medical conditions has been completed. Contact the clinic to see if one is needed.

If you are having difficulty finding a physiotherapist qualified to treat incontinence and Women's Health concerns, you should speak to your family physician. You may contact the Canadian Physiotherapy Association or the American Physical Therapy Association (see Resources listed at the back of the book) for recommendation of a therapist in your area. The Canadian Continence Foundation as well as the National Association For Continence (NAFC) are also excellent sources of information for bladder and bowel health (see Resources for contact information).

Key Points

- Education and appropriate exercise is the cornerstone of a physiotherapy treatment plan.

- Physiotherapists (Canada) and Physical Therapists (USA), use various treatment modalities for normalizing and strengthening muscle tone, as well as to control pain.

- Physiotherapists/physical therapists can offer treatment if you are having difficulty with your pelvic floor exercises or have not seen the results you were expecting.

Did You Know?

According to the Agency for Health Care Policy and Research, U.S. Department of Health and Human Services (former AHCPR, now AHRQ), the least invasive treatment plan should be your first choice; this should be the treatment option with the fewest potential adverse complications. *The panel concluded that behavioral techniques such as bladder retraining and pelvic muscle rehabilitation are effective, low-risk interventions that can reduce incontinence significantly in varied populations.*[20] *Behavioral techniques should be offered to motivated individuals who wish to avoid more invasive procedures or dependence on protective garments, external devices, and medications. Behavioral techniques have few reported side effects and do not limit future treatment options.*[21] *If motivated, most people treated with behavioral techniques show improvement ranging from complete dryness to decreased incontinence episodes.*[22]

Chapter 26: Pharmacological Treatment

Medications are another treatment option for bladder dysfunction. Many women find benefit in a pharmacological approach to relieving symptoms of urge and stress incontinence. It is important to seek the advice of your doctor on the appropriateness of each drug specifically for your symptoms and health status. The following are a list of drugs commonly used for the treatment of female bladder incontinence and their possible side effects. It is important to discuss your current medications with your physician and pharmacist. Some side effects occur due to combinations of pharmaceutical drugs.

Anticholinergic Medication

Anticholinergic drugs are also known as antispasmodic medications. These are used in the treatment of urge incontinence to try to suppress the bladder muscle contraction that produces the strong urge to void. The following medications relax the smooth muscle of the bladder, or relieve muscle spasm in the bladder, and therefore increase bladder capacity. Some examples of anticholinergic medications are:

- Tolterodine (Detrol)
- Oxybutynin (Ditropan)
- Hyoscyamine (Levsin)
- Flavoxate (Urispas)

Long acting forms of Detrol (UniDet) and Ditropan (Ditropan XL) are also available. Detrol and Ditropan are the more frequently used medications for urinary incontinence.

Possible Side Effects

- dry mouth
- blurred vision
- dry skin
- urinary retention
- constipation
- confusion
- drowsiness
- headache
- tachycardia (rapid heart beat)

Tricyclic Antidepressant Medication

Tricyclic antidepressants are another family of drugs used in the treatment of incontinence, however they are not used as frequently as the anticholinergics. These medications affect the brain as well as the bladder. They are effective in improvement of bladder filling as well as helping during the urine storage phase. Some examples of tricyclic antidepressant medications are:

- Doxepin (Sinequan)
- Imipramine (Tofranil)
- Desipramine (Norpramin)
- Nortriptyline (Aventyl)

Possible Side Effects

- dry mouth
- blurred vision
- urinary retention

- constipation
- drowsiness
- tachycardia (rapid heart beat)
- sedation
- tremors
- weight gain
- postural hypotension (sudden drop in blood pressure upon standing)

Hormone Therapy

Some patients suffering with urgency or frequency may find relief with Hormone Replacement Therapy (HRT). HRT medications are available in pill, gel, patch, injection or vaginal cream forms. As well, some doctors offer estrogen in localized treatment forms such as Estring (estradiol vaginal ring) or Vagifem (a vaginal tablet). Vagifem and Estring are time-release forms of estrogen therapy. They are inserted into the vagina and gradually release small doses of hormone over a period of several months. The Estring is sometimes used in combination with a vaginal pessary. Estrogen is used to increase blood circulation and indirectly improve the tone and elasticity in the urogenital structures. While clinical trials have not supported the theory of HRT's usefulness in the treatment of incontinence, HRT does provide good relief for vaginal dryness.

Possible Side Effects

- breast tenderness
- increase in blood pressure
- edema
- nausea
- headache
- blood clot
- possible increased risk of breast and uterine cancer

Drugs that decrease involuntary muscle contractions such as Detrol, Ditropan, Trofranil and Urispas may be prescribed for urge symptoms and urge incontinence. Medications that increase the strength of the muscles around the urethral sphincter such as pseudoephedrine (Sudafed), and estrogen (HRT) may be prescribed for stress incontinence. In the near future we will be seeing promising new drugs for the treatment of stress incontinence. These medications are currently awaiting FDA approval. Combination therapy of these pharmaceutical medications along with proper pelvic floor exercise leads to successful treatment for many women suffering with urinary incontinence.

Key Points

- There are many medications used for the treatment of urinary incontinence. Realize the possible side effects and work with your doctor to find the most suitable medication for you.

- Many women benefit from a pharmacological treatment approach for their bladder symptoms. To improve bladder control, it is important to ensure that proper diet and pelvic floor exercise is combined with drug therapy.

Did You Know?

Incontinence pads, as well as being an ecological concern, may lead to urinary tract infections, skin breakdown and rash.

Chapter 27: Bladder Function Testing

For most women, the reason for incontinence is easy to determine. If your situation is more complex, or your doctor would like to confirm the diagnosis, you may be referred for bladder function tests. One of the most common tests for bladder issues is urodynamic testing. Many procedures are used to evaluate voiding patterns and diagnose dysfunction. Commonly used bladder function tests are as follows:

Urodynamic Studies (UDS)

Urodynamics is a very useful test that gives information about how the bladder is working and if it is properly doing its job. 'Uro' refers to urine or having to do with the urinary system and 'dynamics' refers to a movement against pressure. For urodynamic testing to be performed, catheters (latex tubes) are placed in the bladder, urethra and rectum, and biofeedback sensors may be placed on the pelvic floor muscle. The bladder is filled with water and data is collected. This test studies the filling, storage, and emptying phases of urination as well as tracking the pelvic floor activity during these bladder stages.

This test helps to evaluate pressure in the bladder and how hard it is having to work. The physician may look for data regarding bladder sensitivity, bladder capacity, changes in the volume-to-pressure relationship, bladder compliance, the presence or absence of bladder contractions and urge incontinence. UDS looks at bladder function and how it coordinates with the pelvic floor muscle. During the filling and storage phases your bladder muscle should be relaxed to accommodate the increase in volume, while your pelvic floor muscle should show activity, trying to keep urine in the bladder. During the emptying phase your bladder muscle should be contracting to move urine out, while your pelvic floor should be relaxed to allow urination. If the bladder muscle is contracting when it should be relaxed, this is called an overactive bladder. If you leak urine during this involuntary bladder contraction, it is called urge incontinence. This problem is usually treated non-surgically with physiotherapy, medications, or both.

As the bladder is being filled you will be asked when you have an initial sensation of needing to void. As the bladder continues to be filled, patients are often asked to cough, sneeze or bear down. Any urinary leakage may indicate the presence of stress incontinence. Treatment options for stress incontinence may include medication, surgery, physiotherapy, or a combination of these therapies.

As you bear down, the urodynamic equipment will be measuring your abdominal and bladder pressures. If urinary leakage occurs with very low abdominal pressure, the urethra may not be closing properly. Intrinsic Sphincter Deficiency (ISD) may be the problem. This usually requires surgical correction.

UDS will focus on the flow of urine as well. The total voiding time and voiding volume will be measured, as well as the peak flow rate. This test will inform you if the urine is emptying too quickly or too slowly. If it is too fast, doctors may look for possible scarring that can hold the urethra open. If the flow is too slow, doctors may look for scarring or blockage within the urethra or bladder. Urodynamic data will also determine if one's bladder is holding too much, or not enough urine. Normal bladder capacity is three hundred to six hundred milliliters (ten to twenty ounces). Often the bladder size of women is slightly larger than for men.

Once the bladder flow has been analyzed it is important to look at what was left in the bladder. Catheter insertion is used to fully drain the bladder after uroflowmetry has emptied the bladder. This provides a post-void residual (PVR), a measurement of the amount of urine that remained in the bladder after urinating. PVR may also be measured using ultrasound, or catheter drainage, independent of a full UDS work up. A PVR value of greater than fifty to seventy-five milliliters (one to two ounces) indicates possible bladder outlet obstruction or detrusor muscle dysfunction. This means either something is blocking the urine from flowing out of the bladder, or the bladder is not contracting effectively to empty itself.

Once all of the data is collected, it will be compared to normal values and any deviations can be noted. A graph, or uroflow curve, may be generated to give useful information about the complete urination process. The curve will be studied to note any abnormalities. For example, the peak should occur at approximately 1/3 of the total voiding time. Abnormal uroflow curves will also pick up on detrusor muscle dysfunction or spasms (overactive bladder), abdominal straining during voiding (dysfunctional voiding patterns), and bladder outlet obstruction (BOO). Uroflow testing may be completed independent of UDS for a non-invasive test of urine stream force.

Some larger medical centers offer video urodynamic testing. This procedure provides an x-ray view of the bladder while the urodynamic measurements are being collected. In this way data can be generated while the bladder activity is visualized. Overall, UDS is a very effective and informative tool for analyzing bladder function.

Cystoscopy

Sometimes it is beneficial to actually see the bladder lining. For this a cystoscope may be inserted into the urethra and bladder. This technique offers a visual perspective of the urethral sphincter, the bladder neck, and also the ureters as they drain into the bladder. This approach can locate blockages, growths, polyps and tumors that can then be biopsied. It may also be used to diagnose chronic infection in the bladder and offer information regarding the bladder neck and determine whether it is opening and closing sufficiently.

Standard Tests

Urinalysis, cultures and blood work will likely be tested routinely to rule out possible infection.

Key Points

- Urodynamic testing may be done for patients with bladder symptoms. The results are often very helpful in diagnosing the precise cause of the symptoms. Other tests such as urinalysis, blood work and x-rays are usually done routinely.

- Your physician may also order ultrasound and cystoscopy for a visual perspective.

Did You Know?

Hesitancy refers to having difficulty initiating the urine stream. This can occur if the bladder muscle is underactive, or if the pelvic floor muscle is overactive and not properly relaxing. Staccato peeing is the starting and stopping of the urine flow as you void. This is usually due to the pelvic floor muscle not properly relaxing.

Chapter 28: Surgical Intervention

Surgery is a treatment option used to return the bladder to its proper position within the body. A prolapsed bladder, or the neck of the bladder, can be lifted or tacked-up and then secured in this elevated position. If this is a treatment option that you are interested in, you should discuss surgical options with your physician or surgeon.

It is important to note that while bladder surgery may be very effective in repositioning the bladder or supporting the urethra, it will not address weakened pelvic floor muscles; therefore, strengthening of this region is still very important and may improve the benefits of surgery. It is often recommended that you strengthen your pelvic floor muscle for three months before undergoing surgery. It is in your best interest to strengthen and support all areas of weakness.

Surgery is used for stress incontinence and occasionally for mixed incontinence. Surgical repair is not useful for urge incontinence. Your surgeon will be able to elaborate on why surgery is or is not a good option for your symptoms. Your doctor will need to know if you are planning on having children in the future since this will eliminate some surgical options.

The following are the main categories of surgery for female stress incontinence, with many variations within each.

- Anterior Vaginal Repair (Colporrhaphy)
- Bladder Neck Suspension
- Pubovaginal Sling
- Minimally Invasive TVT Repair

Anterior Vaginal Repair (Colporrhaphy)

The anterior vaginal repair (colporrhaphy) procedure was created for correction of cystoceles. As discussed in Chapter 7: Pelvic Organ Prolapse, a cystocele is the protrusion of the urinary bladder downward and into the vagina. Often the anterior repair (performed vaginally) is done in combination with a bladder neck suspension or pubovaginal sling to address both the prolapsed bladder, as well as urinary incontinence.

Bladder Neck Suspension

If the urethra is not effectively supported, stress incontinence may result. The urethra may become hypermobile and need to be stabilized. The bladder neck suspension procedure will stitch the neck of the bladder onto the pubic bone, ligament or connective tissue beside the pubic bone. This will provide greater support and stability to the bladder neck and urethra during any increase in intra-abdominal pressure such as coughing, sneezing, lifting and straining.

Bladder neck suspensions can be subdivided into categories depending on the area chosen for entry. These techniques can be performed vaginally or through the abdominal wall. If you and your surgeon decide on a vaginal approach, it will be a needle suspension procedure. If entry is made via the abdominal wall, it will be an open or retro pubic suspension.

Common vaginal needle suspension surgeries are;

- Raz
- Stamey
- Modified Pereyra

These vaginal bladder suspension surgeries will attach the urethra onto muscle or connective tissue.

Common abdominal suspension surgeries are;

- Burch
- Marshall Marchetti-Krantz (MMK)

The Burch technique stitches the urethral tissues into the ligaments attached to the pubic bone whereas the MMK stitches the urethral tissues directly into the pubic bone covering. The Burch procedure is used much more frequently than the MMK.

In the past, the vaginal approach has required a shorter hospital stay and recovery period when compared to the abdominal technique. Presently, this is not necessarily the case since the extensive incision required for abdominal access can now be replaced with a laparoscopic approach that uses two or three small incisions. Your surgeon may now perform the Burch procedure laparoscopically, for example. Open abdominal surgery will require a general anaesthetic, several days admission in hospital, possibly self-catheterization post-surgery, and a six-week recovery period. Laparoscopic surgery may be done under a general anaesthetic or epidural, discharge from hospital may be the day of surgery, a catheter is rarely required post-op, and recovery occurs within a few days.

The laparoscopic approach is also used in radio frequency treatment of stress incontinence. This technique uses thermal energy instead of sutures, implants, or injectable bulking agents to suspend the bladder neck. Radio waves are used to warm the lax tissues of the pelvic floor and cause a shrinkage effect in the collagen. This results in a tightening of the soft tissues producing an increased support to the bladder neck.

Pubovaginal Sling

The pubovaginal sling technique takes fascia, or strong connective tissue, from the patient and uses it like a sling or hammock under the bladder neck and urethra for support. The sling is then attached to the covering, or fascia, of the abdominal muscles or the ligaments behind the pubic bones. This surgery is performed vaginally.

The sling material may be harvested from the covering of the abdominal muscle of the patient or removed from a cadaver donor. Some surgeons use a nylon fabric sling instead of fascia.

Minimally Invasive TVT Repair

TVT, tension-free vaginal tape, is used as a minimally invasive surgical alternative. The procedure consists of placing the TVT mesh underneath the mid-urethra to act as a sling. The design of the 'mesh' allows it to be held in place without being anchored. The 'mesh' supports the urethra during sudden movements such as sneezing, coughing and laughing, and the urethra remains closed, preventing the involuntary loss of urine.

In addition to the above categories, some surgeons offer the following procedures when standard surgical options are inappropriate or have been unsuccessful.

- Injection Therapy
- Artificial Urinary Sphincter
- Interstim

Injection Therapy

Some women have stress and urge (mixed) incontinence whether their bladder is full or empty. This is usually accompanied by leakage at unusual times, like simply being in a lying position. This may be due to Intrinsic Sphincter Deficiency (ISD). This may be the result of previous bladder surgery, where nerves may have been cut or damaged, or scar tissue has developed and is pulling the urethra open. In the past this has been a very difficult problem to repair. Injection therapy as a treatment of ISD brings hope for some women. Several types of materials can be used such as the Contigen® Bard® Collagen Implant (taken from the skin of cows) and Durasphere™ (small beads of zirconium coated in carbon). These injectables are introduced through a needle inserted near the urethral sphincter to bulk up the urethral tube (narrowing the diameter of the opening) and assist in better closure. Often several injections are required.

A new area of development is the use of botulinum toxin injections for urinary incontinence. 'Botox' has been studied in the treatment of sphincter malfunctioning in multiple sclerosis patients. Broader application in the treatment of incontinence remains to be seen, subject to future clinical research.

Artificial Urinary Sphincter

On occasion it is necessary to surgically implant an artificial sphincter. This is an inflatable ring that tightens up around the urethra to provide closure. Women must then push on an inflated bulb that sits just below the labial skin, to inflate and deflate the implant. The artificial sphincter is used more frequently in men following prostate surgery, than in women. In men the bulb is located in the testicle.

Interstim

The Interstim device is also surgically implanted but this device is placed near the spine. It is used to stimulate the spinal nerves to trigger relaxation of the nerves sending the messages. This procedure would be considered only if the more simple treatments for an overactive bladder were unsuccessful.

Key Points

- Surgeons use many varieties of procedures to better position the bladder, or bladder neck, within your body. Your surgeon may decide to perform surgery via the abdomen or the vagina. Abdominal surgeries are then further subdivided into open incision and laparoscopic surgery techniques.

- Remember, for the best surgical results; strengthen your pelvic floor muscles pre and post-surgery. Pelvic floor exercises are a good adjunct to surgery.

Did You Know?

For the most successful surgical result, you should never lift more than twenty-five pounds following repair of a prolapse.[23]

Always keep your pelvic floor strong for additional support, and lift with proper body posture.

Chapter 29: Closing Remarks

I would like to thank my wonderful husband and children for all their love, patience, and support. Their constant encouragement and belief in this project gave me the courage to see it through. My deepest appreciation is extended to all my family and friends whose help and advice made this book possible.

Thank you to all the physiotherapists and physical therapists who pioneered this area of Pelvic Floor Muscle Dysfunction and allowed me to learn from their hard work and experience. I am especially thankful to the following therapists who over the years, have taken the time to help me with treatment ideas through documentation, published works, courses and lectures, and many questioning phone calls and e-mails.

- Lynn Assad P.T.: Goffstown, New Hampshire
- Jill Boissonnault M.S.,P.T.: Madison, Wisconsin
- Marla Bookhout M.S.,P.T.: Minneapolis, Minnesota
- Claudia Brown P.T.: Montreal, Quebec
- Dr. Pauline Chiarelli: Australia (Newcastle University)
- Dee Hartman P.T.: Nugeenville, Illinois
- Hollis Herman MS, P.T., O.C.S: Weymouth, Massachusetts
- Janet Hulme M.A.,P.T.: Missoula, Montana
- Pat Lieblich B.P.T.: Vancouver, British Columbia
- Cynthia Markel Feldt M.P.T., A.T.C.: Jacksonville, Florida
- Dianna R. McDonald P.T.: Edmonton, Alberta
- Kathe Wallace P.T.: Seattle, Washington
- Marie-Josee Lord P.T.: Pointe-Claire, Quebec
- Judy Fox P.T.: Ottawa, Ontario

Thank you to the physicians and surgeons who have entrusted me with the treatment of their patients. Their confidence in our Incontinence and Pelvic Pain programs mean more than they will ever know.

My heart-felt thanks go to my patients who have been such a delight to treat. They are the reason I love my work. Their improvements bring me immense joy, and I could not be more proud of their hard work and determination. It was an honor to be part of their treatment programs. I know that they will never take their bladder control for granted again and they deserve every dry day.

Physiotherapist's Viewpoint...

In closing I would like to leave you with one last personal story that had an impact on me. A few months ago my son had one of his kindergarten friends over to play. My son had drawn him a picture of the urinary and gastro-intestinal tracts and was explaining how the "poop and pee comes out" (you can tell what things are discussed in our home). His friend replied with the obvious five-year-old response, "That's gross." My son responded with indignation, "It's not gross. My mom works with kids and mommies who have trouble with peeing and pooing and if I had trouble I'm glad she could help me!" I quietly snuck out of the room to hide my tears of pride.

My appreciation goes to you, the reader, for taking an interest in this very special muscle and its function. I wish you all the very best as you begin your exercise program. It will not always be easy; however, I hope that you have come to the realization that it is time to fight back and regain control. Do not give up—it will take time, but you can win against this challenge. Most of all, please never feel that you are alone with this problem. There are millions of women trying to hide symptoms like yours and there are many health care providers who want to help. I hope this book has the positive effect on your bladder health that is intended. Best of luck to you!

Top 10 Things to Learn from This Book.

1. Incontinence is **not** a normal part of aging.
2. Incontinence is **not** a normal part of childbirth.
3. Incontinence is preventable, treatable and often curable.
4. Do **not** do your exercises on the toilet.
5. You should void every two and a half to four hours, five to nine voids per day and up to one time at night.
6. If you are urinating for less than eight to ten seconds, you probably did not need to void.
7. Daily pelvic floor exercises may prevent incontinence as well as pelvic organ prolapse. Giving good support to your bladder and uterus may prevent the need for future hysterectomy or bladder surgery.
8. It is never too late to start your exercises. The pelvic floor muscle is surprisingly forgiving.
9. Caffeine, artificial sweeteners, alcohol, smoking and excess weight are all contributing factors to incontinence that you have control over.
10. Voiding is a passive event, **never** push. Let your bladder muscle do its job.

References

To ensure that acknowledgement is given to the individuals that have generously shared their invaluable knowledge and information, throughout this book all direct quotations have been distinguished in italics. The remaining references were used as indirect quotations and the information paraphrased. These are not denoted in a special script but do have a numeral corresponding to the appropriate reference listed here. Thank you to the following people whose hard work benefits us all.

1. Is urine leakage keeping you from Sex? Laughing? Golf? Socializing? *The Canadian Continence Foundation*. 2000. Pamphlet.

2 . Consumer Focus: A Survey 1999, National Association For Continence (NAFC), Spartanburg, SC, 1999; 4.

3. "What is Urinary Incontinence?"*MayoClinic.com*. On-line. Internet. June 9 2002. Available <http://www.mayoclinic.com/findinformation/conditioncenters/invoke.cfm?objectid=256654C2-9>.

4. Overactive Bladder, A Medical Condition Many Struggle With Needlessly. *UniDet*. Oct. 2002. Backgrounder.
Decima Research Poll, May 2002.

5. Nitti VW. Clinical Impact of Overactive Bladder. *Rev Urol*. 2002;4(suppl 4):S2-S6.

6. "Center For Bladder Control Innovation, Technology and Care." *Facts About Urinary Incontinence*. On-line. Internet. July 13, 2002. Available <http://www.rizvimd.com/html/incontinence.html>.

7. Nygaard IE, Thompson FL, Svengalis SL, Albright JP. Urinary Incontinence in Elite Nulliparous Athletes. *Obstet Gynecol*. 1994;84(2): 183-7.

8. Shull BL. Pelvic Organ Prolapse: Anterior, Superior, and Posterior Vaginal Segment Defects. *Am J Obstet Gynecol* 1999; 181:6-11.

199

9. *Blueprint for Continence Care in an Assisted Living Setting* published by NAFC, 2000, Spartanburg, SC.
Wagner TH, Hu TW. Economic costs of urinary incontinence in 1995. *Urology* 1998.51(3):355-361.

10. "Center For Bladder Control Innovation, Technology and Care." *Facts About Urinary Incontinence.* On-line. Internet. July 13, 2002. Available <http://www.rizvimb.com/html/incontinence.html>.

11. Grimby A, Milsom I, Molander U, Wiklund I, Ekelund P. The influence of urinary incontinence on the quality of life of elderly women. *Age Ageing.* 1993 Mar;22(2):82-9.

12. *Overview: Urinary Incontinence in Adults, Clinical Practice Guideline Update.* Agency for Health Care Policy and Research (former AHCPR, now AHRQ), Rockville, MD. March 1996. <http://www.ahrq.gov/clinic/uiovervw.htm>.

13. Bump RC, Hurt WG, Fantl JA, Wyman JF. Assessment of Kegel pelvic muscle exercise performance after brief verbal instruction. *American Journal of Obstetrics and Gynecology* 1991;165:322-9.

14. Soifer, S. Paruresis or Shy Bladder Syndrome: The Little Known Urinary Problem. *The Informer.* The Canadian Incontinence Foundation. Winter 2002;3,(1):3.

15. "Center For Bladder Control Innovation, Technology and Care." *Facts About Urinary Incontinence.* On-line. Internet. July 13, 2002. Available <http://www.rizvimb.com/html/incontinence.html>.

16. Benvenuti F, Caputo GM, Bandinelli S, Mayer F, Biagini C, Sommavilla A. *Reeducative treatment of female genuine stress incontinence.* Am J Phys Med. 1987 Aug;66(4):155-68.

17. "Center For Bladder Control Innovation, Technology and Care." *Facts About Urinary Incontinence.* On-line. Internet. July 13, 2002. Available <http://www.rizvimb.com/html/incontinence.html>.

18. Fantl JA, Newman DK, Colling J, et al. *Urinary Incontinence in Adults: Acute and Chronic Management.* Clinical Practice Guideline No.

200

2, 1996 Update. Rockville, MD: U.S. Department of Health and
Human Services. Public Health Service, Agency for Health Care
Policy and Research. AHCPR Publication No. 96-0682. March 1996.
(formerly AHCPR, now AHRQ)

19. Wiener, JS. Incontinence: Is it Inherited? *Quality Care.* National
Association For Continence.2000 Summer;18(3):1.

20. Fantl JA, Newman DK, Colling J, et al. *Urinary Incontinence in
Adults: Acute and Chronic Management.* Clinical Practice Guideline No.
2, 1996 Update. Rockville, MD: U.S. Department of Health and
Human Services. Public Health Service, Agency for Health Care
Policy and Research. AHCPR Publication No. 96-0682. March 1996.
(formerly AHCPR, now AHRQ)

21. Fantl JA, Newman DK, Colling J, et al. *Urinary Incontinence in
Adults: Acute and Chronic Management.* Clinical Practice Guideline No.
2, 1996 Update. Rockville, MD: U.S. Department of Health and
Human Services. Public Health Service, Agency for Health Care
Policy and Research. AHCPR Publication No. 96-0682. March 1996.
(formerly AHCPR, now AHRQ)

22. Fantl JA, Newman DK, Colling J, et al. *Urinary Incontinence in
Adults: Acute and Chronic Management.* Clinical Practice Guideline No.
2, 1996 Update. Roekville, MD: U.S. Department of Health and
Human Services. Public Health Service, Agency for Health Care
Policy and Research. AHCPR Publication No. 96-0682. March 1996.
(formerly AHCPR, now AHRQ)

23. Parker WH, Rosenman AE, Parker R. *The Incontinence Solution.
Answers for Women of All Ages.* 2002; 214.

Other Materials Used

Pauline E. Chiarelli PhD. Womens Waterworks, Curing Incontinence.
2002.

Dianna R. MacDonald. "In Control Again", A Personal Workbook.
1995

Resources

American Physical Therapy Association (APTA)
Section on Women's Health (SOWH)
1111 N. Fairfax Street Alexandria VA 22314
Phone: (800) 999-APTA ext.3230 Fax: (703) 706-8575
Web site: www.apta.org/womenshealth

Bladder Health Council
American Foundation for Urologic Disease
1128N. Charles Street Baltimore, MD 21201
Toll-Free number: (800) 242-2383 Fax: (410) 468-1808
Web site: www.afud.org www. incontinence.org
E-mail: admin@afud.org

The Canadian Continence Foundation
P.O. Box 30, Victoria Branch
Westmount, Quebec, Canada H3Z 2V4
Phone: (514) 488-8379 Toll-free number: (800) 265-9575
Fax: (514) 488-1379 Web site: www.continence-fdn.ca
E-mail: help@continence-fdn.ca

Canadian Physiotherapy Association (CPA)
2345 Yonge Street Suite 410 Toronto, ON, Canada M4P 2E5
Phone: (800) 387-8679 (416) 932-1888
Fax: (416) 932-9708 Web site: www.physiotherapy.ca
E-mail: information@physiotherapy.ca

Endometriosis Association Inc.
8588 North 76th Place Milwaukee, WI 53223
Phone: (800) 992-3636 (414) 355-2200
Fax: (414) 355-6065 Web site: www.KillerCramps.org
E-mail: endo@endometriosisassn.org

Hysterectomy Ed Resources and Services (HERS)
422 Bryn Mawr Ave Bala Cynwyd, PA 19004
Phone: (205) 667-7757
ICEA (International Childbirth Education Association)
PO Box 20048 Minneapolis, MN

ICS (International Continence Society)
Dr. Werner Schaefer Urologische Klinik der RWTH Aacher
Pauwelsstrasse D01500 Aacher, Germany

ICS (Interstitial Cystitis Association)
PO Box 1553 New York, NY 10159-1553
Phone: (212) 979-6057 Web site: www.ichelp.com

IFBD
International Foundation for Functional Gastrointestinal
Disorders
PO Box 170864 Milwaukee, WI 53217
Phone: (414) 964-1799 Web site: www.iffgd.org

IPPC—Incontinence & Pelvic Pain Clinic
(Division of Nova Physiotherapy & Sports Fitness Clinic)
714 Medical Arts Building 233 Kennedy Street
Winnipeg, Manitoba, Canada R3C 3J5
Phone: (204) 982-9178 Fax: (204) 982-9198

IPPS (International Pelvic Pain Society)
Women Medical Plaza
2006 Brookwood Medical Center Drive #402
Birmingham, AL 35209
Phone: (205) 877-2950 Web site: www.ipps.com

National Association For Continence (NAFC)
P.O. Box 8310 Spartanburg, SC 29305
Toll-free number: (800) BLADDER (800) 252-3337
Phone: (864) 579-7900 Fax: (864) 579-7902
Web site: www.nafc.org E-mail: memberservices@nafc.org

NVA (National Vulvodynia Association)
PO Box 4491 Silver Springs MD 20914
Phone: (301) 299-0775 (301) 972-5286
Web site: nva.org

North American Menopause Society
5900 Landerbrook Drive Suite 195 Mayfield OH 44124
Phone: (440) 442-7550
Web site: www.menopause.org E-mail: info.menopause.org

The Simon Foundation for Continence
PO Box 835 Wilmette, IL 60091
Toll-free number (800) 23SIMON (800) 237-4666
Phone: (847) 864-3913 Fax: (847) 864-3913
Web site: www.simonfoundation.org

Index